For EU product safety concerns:
IN TECH d.o.o., Prolaz Marije Krucifikse Kozulić 3, 51000 Rijeka, Croatia,
info@intechopen.com or visit our website at intechopen.com.

Meet the editor

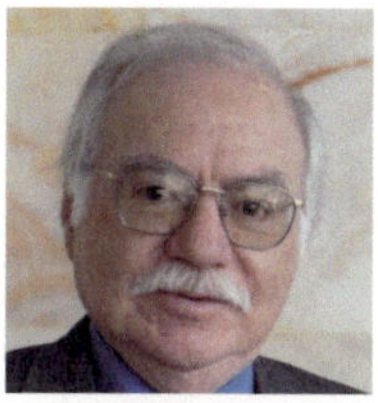

Víctor M. Whizar-Lugo graduated from the Universidad Nacional Autónoma de México and completed his residency in internal medicine at the Hospital General de México, Anaesthesiology and Critical Care Medicine at the Instituto Nacional de la Nutrición in México City. He undertook his fellowship at the Anesthesia Department, Pain Clinic at University of California, Los Angeles, USA. He currently works at the ICU in the Hospital General de Tijuana, ISESALUD. He belongs to the Institutos Nacionales de Salud as an associated researcher. He has 140 publications on anesthesia, pain, internal medicine, and critical care journals/books, has edited three books and given 267 conferences in congresses and meetings of his specialty. He has been a member of various editorial committees in anesthesiology journals, and was chief editor of the journal Anestesia en México. He is currently the editor-in-chief of the Journal of Anesthesia and Critical Care: Open Access. Dr. Whizar-Lugo is the founding director and current president of Anestesiología y Medicina del Dolor www.anestesiologia-dolor.org, a free medical educative program on the internet.

Contents

Preface

Patients submitted to plastic and reconstructive surgery make up a diverse group of people (healthy or with added pathologies) that seek to improve their body image with the ultimate goal of being more competitive in their family, school, work, and social environment. Anesthetizing these people – healthy or not – has become a challenge with many unresolved topics and controversies. Advances in perioperative medicine, especially in anesthesiology, have made it possible to overcome some of these challenges.

In this book, authors from different countries discuss selected topics on anesthesia and plastic and reconstructive surgery. Although some opinions seem to be opposing, all the knowledge is oriented to the safe management of each patient. Preoperative assessment, perioperative monitoring, anesthetic management techniques, complications, post-operative care, and analgesia are some of the topics included in this book.

As the editor, I want to thank each of the authors who contributed to this book and invite colleagues who for various reasons did not finish their manuscripts so that together we can prepare a second project with topics of interest in this field of anesthesiology. It is also right to thank the thousands of patients with whom I have had the fortune to work, as well as distinguished Mexican plastic surgeons, especially Dr. Jaime Campos-León for his confidence and unconditional support of my research and practice in anesthesia for plastic surgery. Finally, it is my pleasure to thank my family for their love and patience, so that I can take part of their valuable time and write down my professional experiences.

Víctor M. Whizar-Lugo MD
Lotus MedGroup
Intensive Care Unit
Hospital General de Tijuana, ISESALUD
Tijuana BC, México

Chapter 1

Anesthesia for Plastic Surgery Procedures

Víctor M. Whizar-Lugo and
Ana C. Cárdenas-Maytorena

Additional information is available at the end of the chapter

http://dx.doi.org/10.5772/intechopen.81284

Abstract

Plastic surgery is currently more popular and available with increasing frequency throughout the world. Its advances are related to progress in anesthesiology. Nowadays, it is possible to operate patients with pathologies that previously did not allow this type of surgery. The developments in perioperative monitoring, pharmacology, prevention of complications, and the wide communication between patients and physicians, as well as the development of surgical units that facilitate a prompt programming and reduce the total costs, have resulted in a logarithmic growth of plastic and reconstructive surgery procedures. Local, regional, or general anesthesia, anesthetic monitoring, or conscious sedation is used routinely, allowing to manage patients as ambulatory or short stay. Deep vein thrombosis and pulmonary embolism remain the most frequent complications, followed by postoperative pain, nausea, and vomiting.

Keywords: plastic surgery, anesthesia

1. Introduction

The current demand for plastic surgery procedures has had a logarithmic growth. The American Society for Aesthetic Plastic Surgery reported that in 2016 in the USA 17.1 million surgical and nonsurgical cosmetic procedures were performed, a figure that indicates a 132% increase since 2000. These procedures represented an expenditure of approximately 16.4 billion US dollars, where breast augmentation is the most popular surgery and the application of Botox is the most performed nonsurgical procedure [1]. Other interesting aspects that have grown around plastic surgery are ambulatory surgery units, short-stay units, and procedures performed in plastic surgeons' medical offices. It is important that anesthesiological care does not decline when surgery is performed in this type of facility and the media and plastic surgeons must be made aware, so they do not minimize the risks of this type of surgery, which from the point of view of the anesthesiologists are medium- and high-risk procedures [2, 3]. Regardless of where the surgery is performed, patient safety should be the primary issue at the time of anesthesia-surgery and during its immediate recovery. To ensure patient safety, there are several guidelines that list the most important points of accomplishment that should be followed in this regard. The published guide from SCARE [4], which emphasizes various points of safety, especially the mechanical and pharmacological prophylaxis of deep venous thrombosis (DVT) and pulmonary thromboembolism (PE). A review of the literature on liposuction complications establishes strict guidelines on lidocaine and epinephrine doses, PE prophylaxis, adequate hydration, and other management recommendations [5].

The advances in plastic surgery have been furthered by the progress in anesthesiology, making it the cornerstone on which the surgical progress has been made. Now, it is possible to carry out prolonged and more elaborate surgeries in patients with concomitant pathologies or with anesthesia risks that some years ago were not possible to achieve with the current safety. The availability of new anesthetics and adjuvant drugs, advances in trans- and postoperative monitoring, as well as the early prevention of complications have facilitated these advances. The list of plastic surgical procedures is very extensive, and anesthesia plays a vital role: from local techniques to neuraxial anesthesia and general inhaled or intravenous anesthesia procedures. The growth of outpatient procedures in cosmetic surgery requires effective anesthetic techniques that allow safe home returns shortly after the surgery is over. It is ideal that no surgical procedure in plastic surgery is performed without the presence of a qualified anesthesiologist.

This chapter serves as an introduction to this book, the most frequent plastic surgery procedures are listed, as well as the anesthesia techniques considered to be the most advanced.

2. Most frequent plastic surgery procedures

It is important that the anesthesiologist be familiar with all surgical procedures to establish an optimal anesthetic approach (see **Graphic 1** and **Tables 1** and **2**). It is also important to keep in mind that the original surgical plan changes frequently; these last-minute modifications obey the wishes of the patient and sometimes the needs that arise during surgery, situations that lead to adjust the original anesthetic plan.

Table 2 lists the most frequent surgical procedures in plastic surgery and relates them to the most used anesthesia techniques, making some important observations in postanesthetic care and evolution. These techniques are the most recommended, being possible to use other alternatives or through combinations of anesthetic methods [6].

In plastic surgery, it is common to combine two or more surgical procedures (breast-abdominoplasty, mommy makeover), which in addition to increasing the risks, prolongs the surgical time, and therefore the anesthetic plan must be adapted to the surgeon's new approach. This fact can be determined before starting anesthesia, and in some patients, it is

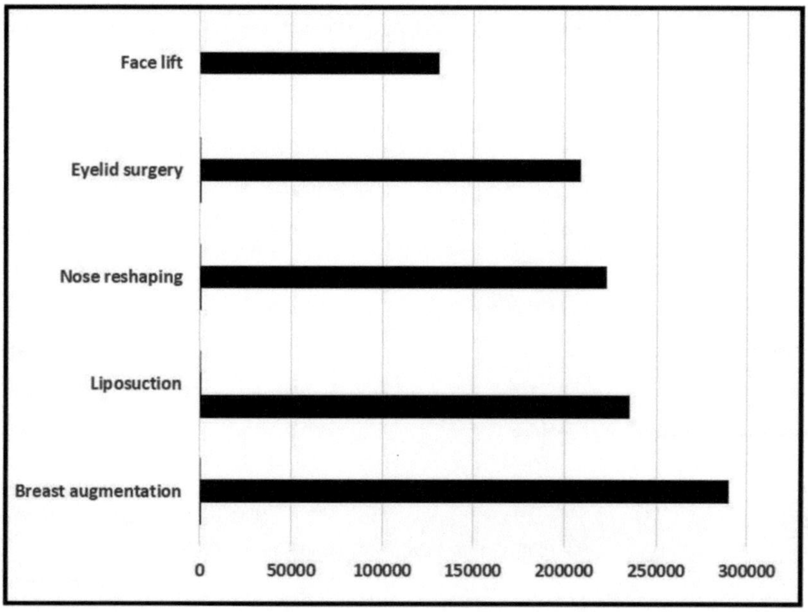

Graphic 1. Most frequent cosmetic surgeries.

Surgery	Women	Men
Breast augmentation	355, 671	
Liposuction	309,692	31,453
Blepharoplasty	166,426	28,678
Abdominoplasty	143,005	
Breast reduction	139,926	
Rhinoplasty		30,174
Gynecomastia		19,124
Hair implantation		18,062

Table 1. Most frequent procedures according to gender [1].

modified during surgery. For example, in a case where breast surgery is combined with abdomen procedures that could otherwise be managed with neuraxial anesthesia, a lumbar spinal anesthesia with hyperbaric local anesthetic and Trendelenburg position could disseminate the blockade up to T3 for breast surgery, which must be performed first, followed by the abdominal procedure [7]. This approach avoids general anesthesia and favors adequate post-operative analgesia with optimal recovery. Combined epidural-spinal anesthesia is another management option in this surgical setting.

Procedures	Anesthesia	Patient stay	Observations
• Facial surgery			
Rhytidoplasty	CS/GA	24 hours	Moderate pain
Coronal	CS/GA	Ambulatory	Fast track
Open rhinoplasty	CS/GA	Ambulatory	Fast track
Rhinoplasty with bone fracture	GA	Ambulatory	Moderate pain
Blepharoplasty	MAC/CS	Ambulatory	Fast track
Otoplasty	MAC/CS	Ambulatory	Fast track
Laser dermabrasion	CS	Ambulatory	Moderate pain
Implants	MAC/CS	Ambulatory	Fast track
Fat grafting, synthetic materials	MAC/CS	Ambulatory	Fast track
• Body surgery			
Breasts or pectorals	PDB/GA	Ambulatory	Moderate pain
Liposuction	SB, PDB, GA, or local	Ambulatory –24 hours	Mild to moderate pain, bleeding, anemia
Torso	PDB /GA	Ambulatory	Moderate pain
Abdominoplasty	SB, PDB/GA	24 hours	Moderate pain, anemia
Breast pexia of inferior segment	PDB/GA	24 hours	Moderate pain, anemia
Buttocks implants	SB/PDB/GA	Ambulatory	Moderate pain
• Limb surgery			
Brachioplasty	PDB/GA	Ambulatory	Moderate pain
Cruroplasty	SB/PDB/GA	Ambulatory –24 hours	Moderate pain
Liposuction	SB/PDB/GA	Ambulatory	Mild pain

CS = conscious sedation; GA = general anesthesia; PDB = peridural block; SB = spinal block; MAC = monitored anesthetic care; fast track = direct access to hospital room.

Table 2. Most frequent procedures in cosmetic surgery.

3. Pre-anesthetic evaluation

"Primum non nocere" is a Latin phrase meaning "first, to do no harm" and is an old statement that has been one of the principal precepts of bioethics for several centuries. This concept is the purpose of pre-anesthetic assessment, which in patients scheduled for plastic surgery should not be any different from that of patients operated of other procedures and should be timely, complete, interdisciplinary, and dynamic. This evaluation is a vital instrument for the medical and nursing team, as well as for the patients and their families since it gives them the opportunity to know the patient and their environment, the reasons that led to surgery, fears of, and above all, to discuss the prejudices and doubts about anesthesia. These patients have peculiarities that make them different; on the one hand, most are healthy people, individuals who do not intend to cure a disease but to improve their self-esteem through better physical appearance. On the other hand, they are extremely demanding patients in terms of perfection in the results and do not tolerate errors or side effects. It is prudent to explain the various anesthetic techniques available for the type of surgery scheduled, as well as the benefits and risks of each anesthetic procedure, especially those attributed to the planned technique. It is also the best time for them to meet the anesthesiologist and become familiar with his/her credentials and experience. These last points are fundamental to gain patient confidence and to diminish their anxiety and the possibility of an eventual legal conflict.

The pre-anesthetic evaluation should be made several days in advance. Regardless of the physical condition of each patient, a complete clinical history and detailed and oriented physical examination are fundamental in the pre-anesthetic assessment. It is essential to determine the physical integrity or possible deterioration of the patient, especially the neurological and cardiopulmonary systems, as well as a detailed analysis of the airway and the spine. The patients must be evaluated regarding their emotional state and their ability to tolerate surgeries with prolonged times and difficult recoveries. Plastic surgery patients are divided into two major categories: healthy patients and patients with one or more systemic pathologies, such as acquired heart diseases, pneumopathies, diabetes mellitus, venous insufficiency, and hyperlipidemia, this last one being the most common. The age at which cosmetic surgery is performed is variable: 35–50 years (45%), 51–64 years (26%), 19–34 (22%), 65 or more (6%), and minors to 18 years (2%) [3].

The healthy patient. Most plastic surgery patients are in good physical shape (ASA 1–2); those with facial surgery are usually more than 50 years old, although cosmetic facial surgery has currently increasing frequency in younger people. Patients who undergo surgery on body segments tend to be younger with purely esthetic goals, but recently there is a growing group of overweight patients who have undergone bariatric surgeries and consult the plastic surgeon seeking corrective procedures for skin excess secondary to excessive weight loss, which should be categorized as unhealthy patients [8, 9]. Patients without apparent comorbidities are potentially healthy people; however, we must be sure that this statement is true. Once the patient has been evaluated by the plastic surgeon, it is recommended that those over 50 years old are also evaluated by an internist and have complete clinical exams according to the surgery plan. These tests should include blood count with platelets, prothrombin time, partial thromboplastin time, INR, complete blood chemistry, and urinalysis. HIV testing is convenient, as well as hepatitis B and C antigens in some patients [3, 6]. Pregnancy test is recommended in women of childbearing age.

During this pre-anesthetic interview, the intake of medications such as nonsteroidal anti-inflammatory drugs (NSAIDs), vitamin E, weight loss medications, contraceptives, herbs, as well as history of illegal drug use or any prescription medicines should be questioned. It is frequent that these "healthy" patients utilize thyroid hormones, antidepressants, benzodiazepines, high doses of vitamins and minerals, as well as herbs, food supplements, and teas that could interact with the drugs used in the perianesthesiological time. Patients underestimate the importance to ingest these products, so it is imperative that both the surgeon and the anesthesiologist emphatically investigate whether patients ingest such products since many of them have anticoagulant, antiplatelet, procoagulant, and arrhythmic or potentiate the effects of anesthetics. Heller et al. [10] found that plastic surgery patients used herbs or supplements in 55% versus the general population 24% ($p < 0.001$). The most used by their patients were chondroitin 18%, ephedra 18%, echinacea 8%, garlic 6%, ginseng 4%, and ginger 4%. Fifty-four percent of the supplements/herbs taken by these patients have pharmacological interference with anesthetic drugs or can affect surgery. In 85% of the cases, patients were not told to stop taking these herbs or supplements before surgery, except for those who ingested ephedra in which 100% of the surgeons indicated their suspension. This study demonstrated the ignorance of physicians regarding the undesirable effects of herbalism in plastic surgery patients. A Mexican study in ambulatory patients [11] found that 65% took ginseng and *Ginkgo biloba* combined, 17.5% ingested garlic, and 5% chamomile tea. **Table 3** lists some herbs and food supplements that should be discontinued 1–2 weeks before the surgery [10–13].

Product	Effect	Product	Effect
Fish oil	Antiplatelet, vasodilation	Kava (*Piper methysticum* root)	Interacts with local anesthetics, barbiturates, increase sedative potency
Garlic (*Allium sativum*)	Antiplatelet	St. John's wort (*Hypericum perforatum*)	Induces cytochrome P450 3A4. Interacts with midazolam, alfentanil, lidocaine, calcium blockers, and serotonin receptor agonists
Alfalfa (*Medicago sativa*)	Anticoagulant Enhances warfarin and ginger effect	Ginseng (*Panax ginseng*)	Anticoagulant
Dong quai (*Angelica sinensis*)	Anticoagulant, antiplatelet	Wild lettuce	Enhances warfarin
Anise	Anticoagulant	Black cohosh	Antiplatelet
Celery	Antiplatelet	Arnica	Anticoagulant
Saffron	Anticoagulant	Papain (papaya proteinase I)	Hemorrhage risk
Boldo (*Peumus boldus*)	Enhances warfarin	Kelp	Anticoagulant
Bromelain	Anticoagulant	*Plantago major*	Coagulant
Castanea sativa	Anticoagulant	Horseradish	Anticoagulant
Onion	Antiplatelet	Licorice root (*Glycyrrhiza glabra*)	Antiplatelet
Clove	Antiplatelet	Red clover	Anticoagulant
Chili pepper (Nahuatl chili)	Antiplatelet	Turmeric (*Curcuma longa*)	Antiplatelet
Ephedra	Vasoconstriction, cardiac infarction, cerebral thrombosis, arrhythmias, hypertension	*Valeriana officinalis*	Increases sedative effect
Echinacea	Promotes infections, allergies, probable hepatotoxic and impaired blood flow	Vitamin E	Antiplatelets
Gingko biloba	Antiplatelet	Asiatic ginseng	Anticoagulant, antiplatelets, hypoglycemic

Table 3. Effects of some herbs and foods.

http://dx.doi.org/10.5772/intechopen.81284

The patient with comorbidities. There are a group of patients who undergo cosmetic surgery and who have one or more added pathologies that warrant a more thorough pre-anesthetic evaluation, which may end up postponing surgical intervention or suspend it indefinitely. Diabetic, hypertensive, cardiac, pulmonary, obese, anemic, hypo-/hyperthyroid, patients with rheumatological diseases, and so on are subjects for consultations with the internist or the appropriate subspecialist to stabilize their concomitant pathologies before programming plastic surgery. It is common for the plastic surgeon to miss some of these systemic pathologies during patient evaluation, so it is mandatory that in the initial anesthesiological assessment a condition that may interfere not only with anesthesia but also with surgery itself or during the healing period should be meticulously researched, such as thrombophilias, hypo-/hyperthyroidism, pheochromocytoma-paragangliomas, lupus, sickle cell disease, drug addiction, and many more. It is the anesthesiologist's role, in conjunction with the surgeon, to refer the patient to the appropriate specialist. Once the patient has been assessed by the internist or a subspecialist, it is advisable to perform a second pre-anesthetic evaluation to be sure that the patient is able to be anesthetized, as well as to know in advance the specialist's recommendations.

Parameters	ASA 1	ASA 2–3	Observations
Clinical history	Yes	Yes	The general and oriented clinical review made by the anesthesiologist anticipates problems such as difficult airway, spinal anomalies, mental alterations, family environment, and possibility of a lawsuit
Physical examination	Yes	Yes	
Specialist consultation	NE	Yes	It is prudent to know the opinion of the geriatrician, pulmonologist, cardiologist, endocrinologist, surgeon, and family therapist in search of polypharmacy, drug interactions, etc.
Electrocardiogram	Only >50 years old	Yes	Arrhythmias, ischemia, growth, or dilatation of heart cavities
Chest X-ray	NE	Yes	Useful in smokers, suspected tuberculosis, neoplasms, emphysema, kyphosis
Echocardiogram	No	R	Compulsory study in patients with severe arterial hypertension, ischemic patients, and patients with dilated cardiomyopathy
Spirometry	No	R	Its usefulness has not been demonstrated; however, it is recommended in chronic pneumopathy and smokers
Blood test	Yes	Yes	Diagnosis of subclinical anemia
Coagulation tests	Yes	Yes	TP, TPT, INR, and bleeding time are mandatory in anticoagulants, hepatocellular damage, severe sepsis, prolonged fasting, and extreme malnutrition
Complete blood chemistry	Yes	Yes	Kidney, hepatocellular, metabolic, and electrolyte evaluation
Urinalysis	NE	Yes	Loss of blood and proteins, changes in urine density
HIV, hepatitis, drugs, pregnancy	R	R	They are requested based on the clinical history and experience data. HIV is prudent for the protection of medical and paramedical personnel

NE = not essential; R = recommendable.

Table 4. Parameters for pre-anesthetic evaluation in plastic surgery [5].

Elderly patients require a more elaborate evaluation, in which it is wise to include the geriatrician. In this group of sick patients, a list that includes all the medications they take should be made, including antihypertensive, diuretic, vasodilator, MAO inhibitors, antidepressants, analgesics, hormones, hypoglycemic agents, vitamins and minerals, etc. The anesthesiologist must be familiar with these drugs and know their possible drug interactions. The usual pre-anesthetic assessment parameters in healthy patients and patients with comorbidities are listed in **Table 4**.

There are patients who should not be operated, and this decision must be made by the anesthesiologist, regardless of the opinion of the patient and his/her surgeon since loss of safety rules leads to catastrophic nonreversible events [14].

Once the anesthetic assessment has been finalized and the best anesthetic plan has been agreed upon and the possible eventualities discussed, the informed consent must be obtained, which as a rule must be signed by the patient, the doctor, and a witness. This document should mention the details of the proposed anesthetic technique, its side effects, and possible complications in a detailed manner. A well-prepared informed consent is a legal document that does not exclude us from a lawsuit, but when it is not done properly, it can be a legal component against the medical team [14–16].

4. Pre-anesthetic medication

The goal of pre-anesthetic medication is to help the patient to arrive to the operating room with sedation, hypnosis, prevention of nausea and vomiting, and with preemptive analgesia. Midazolam and lorazepam are the most commonly used benzodiazepines. Midazolam is more useful in short procedures, although it is less amnesic than lorazepam. There is evidence that melatonin 3–10 mg administered as part of pre-anesthetic medication reduces preoperative anxiety, decreases postoperative pain intensity and opioid consumption, improves postoperative sleep quality, and reduces emergence behavior and postoperative delirium. Also, preoperative melatonin could reduce oxidative stress and anesthetic requirements [17–20]. To prevent nausea and vomiting, it is advisable to use two or more drugs [21]; combining droperidol with dexamethasone is as effective as the combination of ondansetron with dexamethasone. Metoclopramide tends to disappear due to its low clinical effectiveness compared to the new antiemetics. It is convenient to administer omeprazole or ranitidine to reduce the acidity and volume of the gastric secretion. Preemptive analgesia is achieved with the administration of various drugs such as intravenous magnesium, NSAIDs, gabapentinoids, and ketamine to name a few.

5. Anesthesia techniques

In general terms, regional anesthesia techniques are more recommendable than those of general anesthesia since they have less complications and favor a safer recovery, with better postoperative analgesia. In the following paragraphs, several anesthetic procedures are discussed and are related primarily to outpatient surgery since most plastic surgery patients are discharged the same day of their intervention. **Figure 1** shows all the anesthetic techniques that can be used in plastic surgery procedures, a wide range of combinations being possible.

For more details of some anesthetic technique, the reader is referred to the pertinent chapters of this book.

5.1. Conscious sedation

The objective of conscious sedation is to have a patient in a status of restfulness that allows the surgeon to inject local anesthetics and perform their operative procedure with safety and comfort for the patient, while the anesthesiologist is responsible for drug sedation and checking the stability of all systems using conventional monitoring and added BIS. The most frequent surgeries are those of the face and neck, hair implants, liposuction of small areas, dermabrasion with laser, and occasionally breast implants. A clear understanding must be established with the patient and the surgeon about the objectives of conscious sedation: *the technique is not anesthesia,* so the operative pain is managed by the surgeon through the frequent injection of local anesthetics. The opioids used in these cases are a primary part of sedation, not for analgesia. **Figure 2** shows the most important differences between conscious sedation and general anesthesia; note that in conscious sedation the patient maintains the integrity of the airway and its protective reflexes, unlike general anesthesia. There is a tenuous

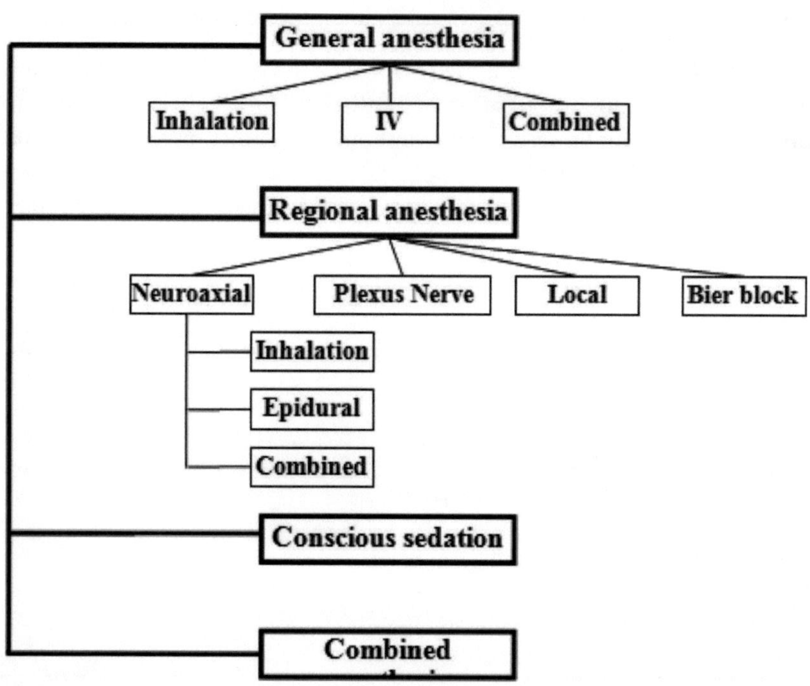

Figure 1. Anesthesia techniques that can be used for plastic surgery.

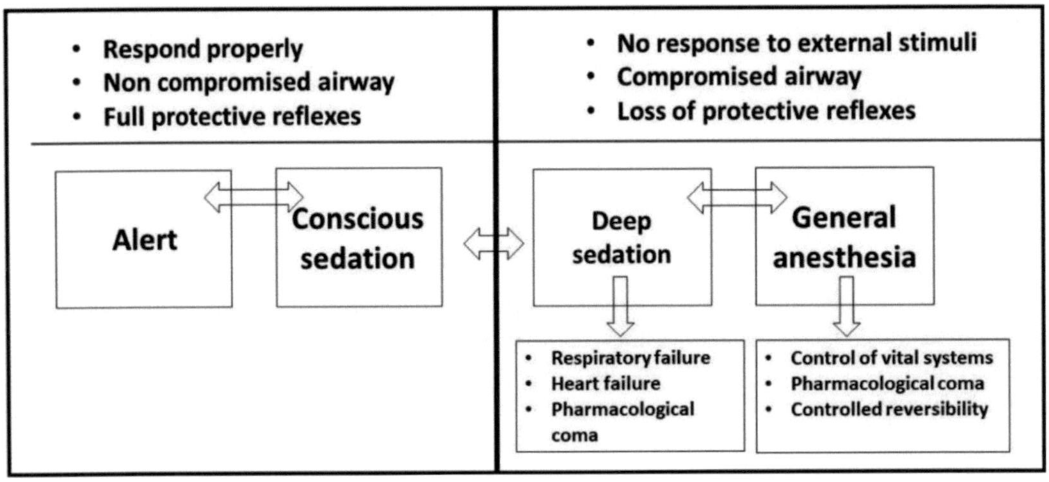

Figure 2. Spectrum of alertness, conscious sedation, deep sedation, and general anesthesia [6].

line of separation between deep sedation and general anesthesia, a situation that often warrants securing the airway and protecting the patient changing the technique to general anesthesia.

There are several types of drugs that are used in conscious sedation: anxiolytics, sedatives, butyrophenones, barbiturates, hypnotics, opioids, and alpha2 agonists (**Table 5**).

The 2018 ASA guidelines for sedation added the following recommendations: patient evaluation and preparation, continual monitoring of ventilatory function with capnography to supplement standard monitoring by observation and pulse oximetry, presence of an individual in the procedure room with knowledge and skills to recognize and treat airway complications, sedatives and analgesics not intended for general anesthesia (e.g., benzodiazepines and

Anesthesia techniques	Opioids	Benzodiazepines	Hypnotics	Alpha-2	Anesthetic gases	Muscle relaxants
TIVA	Fentanyl, remifentanil, alfentanil	Midazolam	Propofol, ketamine	Dexmedetomidine	Nitrous oxide	Vecuronium rocuronium, atracurium
General	Fentanyl Morphine	Midazolam, diazepam	Propofol, ketamine, thiopental	Clonidine, dexmedetomidine	Desflurane Sevoflurane Isoflurane	Vecuronium rocuronium, atracurium
Conscious sedation	Fentanyl Remifentanil Morphine Buprenorphine	Midazolam, lorazepam	Propofol, ketamine, barbiturates	Clonidine, dexmedetomidine	No	No
TCI	Remifentanil	No	Propofol	No	No	No

MAC = monitored anesthetic care; TCI = target-controlled infusion.

Table 5. Anesthesia techniques and examples of usual drugs.

dexmedetomidine), sedatives and analgesics intended for general anesthesia (e.g., propofol, ketamine, and etomidate), recovery care, and creation and implementation of quality improvement processes [22].

5.2. General anesthesia

General anesthesia can be used in all plastic surgery procedures if the location where they have been scheduled fulfills with all safety regulations. This rule should not be violated, especially in medical offices that have been supplemented with an operating room (office based). General anesthesia techniques are used in very short procedures, in patients who reject regional techniques, and as a complement to regional anesthesia when this is not sufficient. In prolonged surgeries of more than 3 hours, it is prudent to avoid the use of general anesthesia when this is possible to prevent risks and undesirable side effects such as nausea, vomiting, oropharyngeal discomfort secondary to the endotracheal tube or laryngeal mask, DVT, PE, postoperative pain, postoperative delirium, and so on. The costs of general anesthesia, although not a definitive factor, do influence the anesthesiological decision, particularly when the procedures are very long. The selection of patients for general anesthesia must be meticulous and exclude those cases with associated pathologies: angina, recent history of cardiac infarction, cardiomyopathies, uncontrolled arterial hypertension, terminal renal failure, sickle cell anemia, patients in need of organ transplantation, active multiple sclerosis, severe chronic obstructive pulmonary disease, difficult airway, malignant hyperthermia, abuse of illegal drugs, dementia, myasthenia gravis, obstructive sleep apnea, and etcetera [23, 24]. In some of these associated pathologies, it is possible to perform plastic surgery; however, precautions must be taken for each disease due to potential complications.

When general anesthesia has been chosen, the drugs to be used should be selected for safety and anesthetic efficacy, in accordance with the surgical location. The ideal technique does not exist, but it must be ensured that it is with a gentle and rapid induction, with adequate operative conditions, with great hemodynamic stability and fast recovery, without side effects, with good control of postsurgical acute pain, with emesis, and with preventive management of postoperative chronic pain. There is not enough evidence to select one drug over another; however, the halogenated anesthetics desflurane, sevoflurane, and isoflurane have demonstrated their versatility in outpatients with a minimum of differences that do not impact the transoperative evolution or the recovery of patients [23, 25]. It is convenient to avoid nitrous oxide due to the high incidence of postoperative nausea and vomiting. Propofol, ketamine, and remifentanil have been widely accepted in this field, each of them having certain advantages. The combination of propofol-ketamine has been studied by Friedberg [25] and proposed as an alternative to inhalational anesthesia.

5.3. Regional anesthesia

Regional anesthesia has had an increasing resurgence since it favors several positive aspects in the trans, operative period, and in the recovery phase. Local anesthesia is performed by the plastic surgeon in cases of minimal invasion such as blepharoplasty, chin implant, and some small liposuction among other procedures. Neuraxial anesthesia, especially spinal anesthesia, has been favored by its advantages (**Table 6**). Capdevila and Dadure [26] consider that the various techniques of regional anesthesia, including spinal anesthesia, are superior to general anesthesia in limiting adverse effects and readmissions to the hospital, with better control of postoperative pain [27]. In the following paragraphs, subarachnoid and epidural block are described, although the latter is less used because it has more possibilities of undesirable effects.

5.3.1. Neuraxial anesthesia

Neuraxial blocks offer several advantages over general anesthesia, as shown in **Table 6**. The decrease in metabolic response to trauma, postoperative analgesia, lower incidence of nausea and postoperative vomiting, and their low costs are just some of these advantages.

Subarachnoid anesthesia. Spinal anesthesia satisfies the current requirements of efficacy and safety that allow early home discharges. It produces an optimal anesthetic status, is easy to administer, has a quick start, and has a low cost. The recovery of the motor and sensory block can be manipulated according to the operative time when local anesthetics and adjuvant drugs available for clinical use are used rationally. Side effects are easy to manage, and complications are rare [27, 28]. There are multiple studies in various clinical scenarios that demonstrate the benefits of spinal anesthesia using small spinal needles (gauge 26–29), with cutting or pencil tip in patients undergoing ambulatory or short-stay surgical procedures [29–31]. Spinal anesthesia versus desflurane [32] in ambulatory patients demonstrated, in addition to a lower cost with spinal anesthesia, that 50% of those who received general anesthesia required postoperative analgesia versus 0% in those who were managed with subarachnoid block. Another research [33] found no cost difference between both techniques and showed that administering spinal anesthesia consumes more time (18 ± 8 min vs. 10 ± 3 min), with more time in the postanesthesia recovery room (123 ± 51 min vs. 94 ± 48 min). The antiemetic requirements were higher in general anesthesia (8% vs. 14%), while the need for analgesics in the immediate postsurgical period was only 25% in those who were treated with spinal anesthesia versus 75% in the group treated with general anesthesia. Carrada et al. [34] compared three spinal needles,

	General	Sedation	Peridural	Spinal	Combined	PNB*
Bleeding	++++	++	++	++	+ a ++	+ a ++
DVT/TEP risk	High	Low	Low	Low	Low	Low
Anesthetic toxicity	Remote	Remote	Feasible	Very remote	Feasible	Feasible
Hypoxia PO	Frequent	Possible	Possible	Possible	Possible	Possible
Analgesia PO	No	No	Yes	Yes	Yes	Yes
Technical difficulty	Remote	No	Possible	Possible	Possible	Frequent
Cognitive disorders	++++	++	++	++	+	No
Cost	High	High	Medium	Low	High	High

*Peripheral nerve block.

Table 6. Advantages and disadvantages of the different techniques in anesthesia for plastic surgery.

Atraucan 26, Quincke 26, and Whitacre 27, in young patients and found a very low incidence of post-dural-puncture headache (PDPH), without statistical significance among the three groups. In plastic surgery spinal anesthesia is used for surgical procedures involving the abdomen, perineum, and lower extremities. Any surgical procedure below the sixth dermatome is viable to be managed with spinal anesthesia. In some ambulatory plastic surgery procedures, it is possible to use lumbar subarachnoid block with diffusion up to T2–T3 dermatomes, for breast surgery and chest liposuction [7, 8, 27, 28]. **Tables 7** and **8** list cosmetic surgery procedures and the doses of local anesthetics in which it is possible to use subarachnoid anesthesia, including the cases mentioned up to T2–T3 dermatomes. In some circumstances, it is prudent to use the combined epidural-intrathecal technique to ensure enough duration in some procedures [7].

When the scheduled plastic surgery is longer than 2 hours, it is advisable to add an adjuvant drug such as clonidine in doses of 75, 150–300 μg, fentanyl 12.5–25 μg, or sufentanil 5–10 μg [27, 35]. It is imperative to consider that the operative time could be longer than the surgeon's estimate since there are many "dead times" that prolong the total time required to complete the surgery. **Table 9** shows the possibilities of mixtures of local anesthetic plus adjuvants according to the expected surgical times. Note that the possibility of 1-hour surgeries is included, which is rare in this field: scar reviews, small areas of liposuction, perineal plasties, etc. The combination of procaine + clonidine + fentanyl is excellent. Low doses of local anesthetic of the family pipecoloxylidide (PPX) (bupivacaine, mepivacaine, ropivacaine, and levobupivacaine) are good but usually last longer, and in a very busy environment, they could prolong the time of home discharge. For surgeries lasting up to 2 hours, local anesthetic PPX in low doses and added adjuvant drugs are an ideal combination.

The local hyperbaric anesthetics have an ampler intrathecal cephalic diffusion than the isobaric ones, which is useful in the operative procedures in high dermatomes (upper abdomen and thorax). On the other hand, isobaric local anesthetics are better in the pelvis and lower extremities. Opioids, especially fentanyl, improve the quality of anesthesia without affecting recovery.

Surgery	Spinal		Epidural		APEC	
	Anesthetic	Adjuvant	Anesthetic	Adjuvant	Anesthetic	Adjuvant
Liposuction	L, B, LB, R, M	C, F	L, R, B, LB, M	C, F	L, R,B, LB, M	C, F, S
Liposculpture	B, LB, R, M	C, F	L, R, B, LB, M	C, F	L, R,B, LB, M	C, F, S
Buttocks implants	L, B, LB, R, M	C	L, B, LB, R, M	C	L, R,B, LB, M	C, F, S
Calf implants	L, B, LB, R, M	C	L, B, LB, R, M	C	L, R,B, LB, M	C, F, S
Breast with liposuction	B, LB, R, M	C, F	L, R, B, LB, M	C, F	L, R,B, LB, M	C, F, S
Breast	—	—	L, R, B, LB, M	no	—	—

APEC = combined peridural-spinal anesthesia; L = lidocaine; B = racemic bupivacaine; LB = levobupivacaine; R = ropivacaine; M = mepivacaine; C = clonidine; F = fentanyl; S = sufentanil.

Table 7. Frequent procedures and regional techniques in ambulatory cosmetic surgery [20].

Surgery	Concentration of local anesthetic and total dose in mg			
	Ropivacaine (0.75%)	Levobupivacaine (0.75%)	Bupivacaine (0.5–0.75%)	Lidocaine (2%)
Liposuction	10–22.5	7.5–18	7.5–15	50–100
Liposculpture	10–22.5	7.5–18	7.5–15	50–100
Buttocks implants	15	10	10	100
Calf implants	15	10	10	100
Breast with liposuction	22.5	18	18	No

*Local hyperbaric anesthetics. The addition of adjuvants will depend on the expected time of surgery.
Lumbar approach, with local hyperbaric anesthetic. With or without high lumbar epidural catheter.

Table 8. Outpatient plastic surgery procedures and doses of intrathecal local anesthetics* [20].

Approximate duration	Drugs and recommended doses	Observations
Surgery up to 1 hour	Lidocaine 30–100 mg	The use of lidocaine tends to disappear due to the possibility of local neurotoxicity
	Lidocaine 30–50 mg + clonidine 75 μg	
	Lidocaine 30–50 mg + fentanyl 25 μg	
	Bupivacaine 5–7.5 mg + clonidine 75 μg or fentanyl 25 μg	Local anesthetics of the PPX family used in low doses tend to replace the use of lidocaine in brief procedures
	Levobupivacaine 5–7.5 mg + clonidine 75 μg or fentanyl 25 μg	
	Ropivacaine 7.5–10 mg + clonidine 75 μg or fentanyl 25 μg	
	Procaine 100–200 mg + clonidine 75 μg or fentanyl 25 μg	Its short duration improves with the addition of adjuvants
Surgery from 1 to 2 hours	Bupivacaine 10–15 mg + clonidine 150 μg and/or fentanyl 25 μg	The duration of the average doses of PPX local anesthetics is prolonged with the addition of clonidine in a dose-dependent manner
	Levobupivacaine 10–15 + clonidine 150 μg and/or fentanyl 25 μg	
	Ropivacaine 15–20 + clonidine 75 μg and/or fentanyl 25 μg	
Surgery greater than 2 hours	Bupivacaine 15–20 mg + clonidine 150–300 μg and/or fentanyl 25 μg	High doses of clonidine favor spinal anesthesia that can reach 3–5 hours of surgical anesthesia, with excellent postoperative analgesia
	Levobupivacaine 15–20 mg + clonidine 150–300 μg, and/or fentanyl 25 μg	
	Ropivacaine 20–30 mg + clonidine 150–300 μg and/or fentanyl 25 μg	

Table 9. Local anesthetics and coadjuvant drugs in spinal anesthesia [20].

Subarachnoid anesthesia in plastic surgery procedures can be done with a single injection, with or without adjuvant drugs, usual doses, low doses or high doses, or combined with extradural anesthesia. The single injection with spinal anesthesia with mono-dose is an easy, safe, and economic technique that produces a deep anesthetic and motor block, with a low incidence of failure and undesirable side effects. It is the procedure most used in short- and medium-length surgeries, being able to be used in some prolonged procedures such as abdominoplasties with or without breast surgery. It is recommended to use small spinal needles G26, G27, and G29, with blunt tip, cutting tip, or special cutting tip. Low doses of long-acting local anesthetics play an important role in outpatients [27, 28]. A comparative study with 6 mg of hypobaric bupivacaine (0.5% in 1.2 mL) versus 6.1 mg of almost hypobaric bupivacaine (0.18% in 3.4 mL) had similar effects on the anesthetic level, duration of sensory, and motor block [36]. Dosage of 6 mg of bupivacaine versus 7.5 mg of bupivacaine [37], both doses added with 25 μg of fentanyl, has similar results in terms of diffusion, duration, and regression of the sensory block. Doses between 5 and 8 mg of ropivacaine, levobupivacaine, or bupivacaine provide up to 150 minutes of intrathecal anesthesia, enough time for most outpatient procedures in cosmetic surgery, time that can be prolonged with the addition of 150–300 μg of spinal clonidine up to 3–5 hours. The most used doses vary from 10 to 15 mg of hyperbaric bupivacaine, being possible to increase these doses up to 20–25 mg in special cases. Drowsiness, bradycardia, and hypotension of easy control are the most frequent effects.

Epidural block. The epidural block is indicated in the same type of surgery as spinal anesthesia, although there are some important considerations: (a) The doses of local anesthetic should be monitored since in prolonged procedures or those in which local anesthetics are injected by the surgeon, there is the possibility of systemic toxicity when the recommended total doses are exceeded or in a delayed form by absorption from the injection site. It is important to remember that lidocaine metabolites have a neuro- and cardiotoxic systemic effect. (b) The initial epidural test dose with local anesthetic should always be repeated before applying a booster dose, especially when the patient has been repositioned in the surgical table (a frequent situation in plastic surgery), due to the possibility that the epidural catheter may be moved from its initial epidural placement [38]. (c) Apparent or unnoticed accidental dural puncture and subsequent PDPH is a possibility, even in the most experienced hands. (d) The quality of the anesthesia is not as deep as that produced by the subarachnoid injection. On the other hand, extradural blockade has the advantage of being able to be prolonged during several days for postoperative analgesia in patients who require it. Ropivacaine, levobupivacaine, and racemic bupivacaine, added with clonidine, fentanyl, sufentanil, or morphine, are recommended, according to the expected surgical time. Hafezi et al. [39] compared 24 cases of tummy tuck-liposuction performed with general anesthesia versus 371 patients managed with epidural block and found a case with PE in the first group (4%). No cases of DVT/PE were found in the second group. The authors attribute this finding to the differential blockade with epidural bupivacaine that allows transoperative movements of the lower extremities which could be a prophylactic factor of DVT and resultant PE.

Combined subarachnoid-epidural anesthesia. In cases with prolonged surgeries, it is advisable to place an inert lumbar epidural catheter with a cephalad direction to guarantee that in case surgery is prolonged, the anesthetic time can be amplified [7]. When this technique is used, an epidural test dose should always be injected since it is possible that the catheter may migrate to the subdural or subarachnoid space, or there may be migration of the anesthetic or adjuvants through the previous dural orifice [38].

Contraindications of neuraxial anesthesia. Contraindications of neuraxial anesthesia have been modified and are currently reduced to well-defined situations as shown in **Table 10**. In addition to these general contraindications, there are few situations in which it is not appropriate to use spinal anesthesia in this group of patients. Patients planning a flight in the days immediately following their surgery should not receive spinal anesthesia, since pressure changes in the aircraft cabins could facilitate the exit of cerebrospinal fluid through the hole in the dura mater. Patients who live far from the site where they are anesthetized and who are not willing to return to the surgical location should not be managed with spinal anesthesia since in both instances the patient could develop PDPH. Although this is not likely to occur, the mere fact of not being able to return to the place where they were anesthetized could imply that they should be treated by other anesthesiologists in their place of origin, which could facilitate unnecessary legal medical problems [28].

Complications of neuraxial anesthesia. Although spinal anesthesia started with a complicated case of PDPH more than 100 years ago, it has been shown to be safe in outpatient and non-ambulatory patients. Its complications include (a) The immediate ones that include failure of the procedure, total spinal anesthesia due to high doses, direct trauma to the spinal nerves, and injury to the conus medullaris or the spinal cord. Arterial hypotension and bradycardia are frequent, especially in young patients, which can progress to cardiac arrest if not managed in a timely manner. In 1988, Caplan [40] drew attention by publishing 14 cases of unexpected cardiac arrest during spinal anesthesia, an event that continues to occur with an incidence as variable as 1.3–18 cases in 10,000 or 6.4 ± 1.2 in 10,000 spinal anesthesia. The decrease in preload volume promotes bradycardia mediated by three different reflex mechanisms: decrease in the frequency of the cardiac pacemaker due to a decrease in the distension of its fibers, decrease in the trigger pressure of the baroreceptors of the right atrium and the vena cava superior, and the involvement of the Bezold-Jarisch reflex when the receptors of the left

Absolute

- Patient rejection
- Severe coagulation disorders
- Cutaneous sepsis at the possible puncture site

Relative

- Septicemia
- Pre-existing diseases of the central nervous system
- Multiple sclerosis
- Spina bifida
- Neoplasms
- Derived hydrocephalus
- Anticoagulation
- Thrombocytopenia and thrombasthenia
- Severe anatomical alterations
- Conditions dependent on the preload
- Aortic stenosis
- Obstructive hypertrophic cardiomyopathy
- Travel by plane in a postanesthetic medium

Table 10. General contraindications for neuraxial anesthesia.

ventricle are stimulated by the fall of the ventricular volume. The vagal response to the preload decrease produces even more bradycardia that can be accompanied by nausea, vomiting, diaphoresis, and syncope, which can progress to cardiovascular collapse and death. (b) Later complications occur when the anesthetic block has ended and within a month of evolution: transient irritation syndrome of posterior roots, PDPH. Other uncommon complications are bleeding, neuroinfections, arachnoiditis, and low back pain. Complications of epidural anesthesia are due to inadequate technique: perforation of the dura, PDPH, injection of drugs into extradural veins with systemic manifestations of acute toxicity, inadequate anesthesia, rupture or knot in the catheter, retention of the epidural catheter, local infections, etc.

Peripheral nerve blocks. This type of regional anesthesia is rarely used in plastic surgery since most of these surgeries are bilateral. However, some blockages such as thoracic paravertebral, intercostal approaches have been recommended in breast surgery because, in addition to anesthesia, they produce excellent postoperative analgesia, reduction in postoperative opioid consumption, less nausea and vomiting, as well as decrease in length of hospitalization time. Interfacial plane blocks, although they do not produce adequate surgical anesthesia, are recommended techniques for postoperative analgesia. Some of these blocks are discussed later and in other chapters of this book.

6. Anesthesia for most common plastic surgeries

Without pretending to exhaust the topic, this section reviews the usual anesthesia techniques for most common procedures in plastic surgery: breast implants, liposuction, abdominoplasty, rhytidoplasty, combined cosmetic surgeries, and fat transfer.

6.1. Breast implants

Breast implant surgery occupies the first place among cosmetic surgery procedures in the USA, and it is likely that the same happens in other countries. Most patients are healthy, but there are some cases of women with breast reconstruction and implants who have a history of surgery for breast cancer. Several anesthesia techniques have been described for this procedure such as general inhaled or intravenous anesthesia, cervicothoracic epidural block, intercostal blocks, facial plane blocks, and tumescent injection with lidocaine. The advantage of regional techniques is that it produces less nausea, vomiting, postoperative pain, and has a lower cost [41, 42]. Cervicothoracic epidural block with approach in C7–T1 and T3–T4, with lidocaine 1%, ropivacaine 0.75%, bupivacaine 0.5%, or levobupivacaine 0.5% (8–12 mL), produces enough anesthesia with better postoperative analgesia than general anesthesia. A single dose of one of the mentioned local anesthetics is adequate in most cases, and when required, a second epidural dose must be injected through the epidural catheter. Epinephrine 1:80,000 can be added (except when ropivacaine is used) to prolong duration of local anesthetics. The most common side effects include transient elevation of blood pressure with tachycardia, tremor, nasal congestion, and nausea. Hypotension and difficulty breathing are rare [42]. It is also possible to use paravertebral or intercostal nerve blocks. Since Blanco et al. described ultrasound-guided interfacial plane blocks for postoperative breast analgesia; modifications to the initial technique have been published [43–45]. Interfacial blocks score over traditional regional anesthetic procedures as they have no risk of sympathetic blockade, intrathecal or epidural spread which may lead to hemodynamic instability, and prolonged hospital stay [44]. These blocks are not an alternative to general anesthesia, epidural anesthesia, or paravertebral blocks since they do not produce adequate regional surgical anesthesia. However, they can be supplemented with intravenous sedation techniques, general anesthesia, or neuraxial anesthesia. Postoperative pain not only involves the breasts; it can extend to the sternum, lateral aspect of the thorax, armpits, and middle back, being more severe when the implants are submuscular. Postoperative pain can be managed with NSAIDs such as parecoxib, ibuprofen, ketoprofen, ketorolac, or diclofenac combined with low doses of opioids. Tramadol is recommended because of its dual mechanism of analgesic action. Methocarbamol can be associated with the previous scheme. Some investigators have found adequate analgesia with the continuous or intermittent administration of local anesthetics through catheters implanted during surgery [46, 47]. It has not been defined if paravertebral blocks decrease the incidence of chronic postoperative pain in breast surgery [48].

6.2. Surgeries for abdominal contour

The evaluation of candidates for abdominal contour surgery allows patients to be classified according to the possibilities of surgery taking in consideration the skin, fat, and muscles. This group includes liposuction, abdominoplasty, abdominal muscle repair, and various combinations that lengthen the operative time such as a 360° liposuction and mommy makeover.

Liposuction. Liposuction is the second most common procedure in plastic surgery, and it is perhaps the one with the highest morbidity and mortality [49]. Liposuction consists in removing fat from unwanted areas to build and improve contour. It can be performed in most subcutaneous fat deposits, being more frequent in the abdomen, hips, waist, torso, neck, and extremities. In men, it is usually done also in the pectoral region. The selection of patients is a determining factor since there are people who want to sculpt their silhouette because they have failed in weight loss and are looking for massive liposuction as a fast track to their false expectations of a suitable silhouette without taking into consideration that this procedure is not an alternative for the management of obesity. The pre-anesthetic assessment should be meticulous and must reject patients with moderate or severe cardiomyopathies or pneumopathies and those with thrombophilia or a history of pulmonary embolism. It is advisable not to associate liposuction with non-plastic procedures such as gynecological surgery. Surgeon and anesthesiologist must make a comprehensive management plan to meet the goals of patients, when possible. **Figure 3** is a plasticine model developed by one of our patients to inform the surgeon of her esthetic goals with liposuction and fat gluteal grafting.

There are two types of liposuction: the dry technique and the tumescent one. The latter is defined as the removal of subcutaneous fat under anesthesia infiltrated with large volumes of saline solution added with epinephrine and a local anesthetic, usually lidocaine. The original definition excludes the use of another type of anesthesia, whether it is neuraxial or general, as well as the fact that it is done without the presence of an anesthesiologist. However, currently

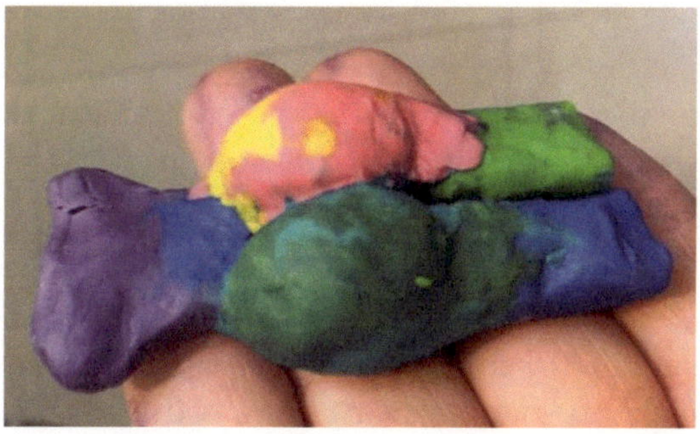

Figure 3. Plasticine model made by the patient to accurately show us the shape and size that she wants for her buttocks.

this type of liposuction is frequently done with epidural block, with spinal anesthesia, or with general anesthesia, in addition to infiltration with Klein's solution (50 mL of 1% lidocaine solution (500 mg), 1 mL of 1:1000 epinephrine (1 mg), 1000 mL of 0.9% saline, and 12.5 mL of 8.4% NaH_2CO_3 solution (12.5 mEq)) [50]. This type of anesthesia involves a dose of lidocaine 35–55 mg/kg of body weight and added epinephrine to achieve concentrations of 0.25–1.5 mg/L, without exceeding total adrenaline total dose of 50 μg/kg. These high doses make it obligatory to perform these procedures in surgery rooms that have all the facilities for monitoring, cardiac resuscitation, ventilatory support, and, always, recovery area under the care of an anesthesiologist. It is an apparently low-risk procedure, which can be complicated by systemic toxicity from local anesthetics, hypothermia, fat embolism, electrolyte imbalances with fluid overload, and/or acute anemia [51, 52]. One of the limitations during cosmetic surgery, especially during tumescent liposuction, is the total dose of the local anesthetic. For this reason, it is advisable not to combine liposuction with other procedures that require the injection of local anesthetics as the maximum dose of these drugs can be exceeded. There is no informed agreement in the literature on what is the top dose of lidocaine; the literature written by dermatologists and plastic surgeons mentioned 55 mg/kg of weight [50, 52–54], whereas the literature that comes from investigations carried out by anesthesiologists mentions 5 mg/kg of weight. In Europe, it is considered safe to use a total of 200 mg of lidocaine without epinephrine, and up to 300 mg is allowed in the United States of America. When epinephrine is added, the lidocaine dose in both regions is 500 mg. Epinephrine 1:200,000 reduces absorption of subcutaneous lidocaine by 50% and intercostal, epidural, and brachial in 20–30% [55]. PPX local anesthetics should never be used in tumescent liposuction. There is no agreement on the best anesthetic technique for liposuction, whether it is the modality under local anesthesia with the Klein solution or with general anesthesia or neuraxial block. With both procedures deaths have been reported [49, 56, 57], and the reports are not completely reliable.

The total volume of fat removed should not exceed 5 L in a single intervention or not be greater than 5% of body weight [58, 59]. Higher volumes increase the risk of complications, especially hypovolemia due to bleeding and acute hydro-electrolytic alterations. Another topic of interest in the management of these patients is the replacement of fluids during the trans-anesthetic period; Trott et al. [60] recommended the following scheme: (a) liposuction of small volumes (<4 L of aspirate) = maintenance liquids + the volume of the injected subcutaneous solution and

(b) liposuction of large volumes (aspirated ≥4 L) = maintenance liquids + the volume of the solution injected +0.25 mL intravenous crystalloids per mL of aspirate extracted after 4 L. These authors emphasize that this fluid replacement guide does not replace a good clinical criterion and communication between the surgeon and the anesthesiologist is always fundamental. The goal is to maintain a normal intravascular volume with a postanesthetic hematocrit above 30% and albumin levels above 3 g.

The so-called 360° liposuction has become fashionable. It is a procedure that combines liposuction of the entire truncal midsection to accomplish a complete curvier contour figure from every angle. It can be combined with dermolipectomy, with plication of the rectus abdominis muscle, and with or without umbilicoplasty or gluteal fat grafting [61, 62].

Abdominoplasty. Surgery of the abdominal wall usually involves resection of skin excess and can be done with or without liposuction (lipoabdominoplasty) and with or without plication of the rectus abdominis muscle [63]. The most common patients include those that have had multiple pregnancies or patients that have lost a lot of weight either by dieting and exercise or after bariatric procedures.

Mommy makeover. The combination of two or more simultaneous cosmetic surgeries has become fashionable, particularly breast surgery and tummy tuck [64]. In our plastic surgery group, the most usual combination is breast-abdominoplasty, liposuction, and gluteal lipoinjection. For abdominal body contour surgeries (liposuction, abdominoplasty, and mommy makeover), we prefer spinal anesthesia with lumbar approach, taking the block up to T4. Due to the length of the procedure, it is prudent to use some adjuvant that prolongs the anesthetic time up to 4–5 hours. Bupivacaine 0.5% 15–20 mg added with clonidine 150–300 μg is strongly recommended [27]. Ropivacaine or L-bupivacaine can also be used. The combination of two or more surgeries of the body contour is now safe, having overcome the complications of the individual procedures. It is vital to establish measures to prevent DVT, PE, infections, and postoperative pain, to name a few [64].

Rhytidoplasty. Cosmetic facial surgery involves several procedures, some of which are performed under local anesthesia injected by the plastic surgeon [65]. Surgeries in which the intervention of the anesthesiologist is required involve generally prolonged interventions, in healthy patients or with added pathologies, in which plastic surgeons request the support of an anesthesiologist to guarantee suitable transoperative care. Local anesthesia (subcutaneous and nerve blocks) combined with conscious sedation is the technique most used in our clinic [6]. Pre-anesthetic medication is the key to have a patient in optimal conditions: sedation, anxiolysis, and preventive analgesia. We recommend 10 mg oral melatonin, 2 mg sublingual lorazepam, and 0.1–0.2 mg of oral clonidine administered 1 hour before taking the patient to the operating room. A low dose of an opioid (morphine 5–10 mg, fentanyl 25–50 mg, buprenorphine 150–300 μg) may be given. To prevent nausea and vomiting, it is recommended to add dehydrobenzoperidol 1.25 mg, dexamethasone 4–8 mg, or any of the 5-HT3 receptor antagonists or setrons (ondansetron, granisetron, dolasetron, and palonosetron). For maintenance, one or more drugs may be used in infusion: ketamine-midazolam, ketamine-propofol, and dexmedetomidine with or without low doses of opioid [6, 25, 66]. These drugs should be infused and diluted, in separate i.v. bags solutions to adjust the sedative, analgesic, or dissociative dose with appropriate doses of each drug to maintain adequate sedation

(Ramsay 3–4, BIS 80–70). Nasal oxygen should be administered throughout the procedure to maintain normal O_2 saturation. The patient must be monitored, as well as corneal protection to avoid abrasive injuries. It is mandatory that the surgical group looks out frequently the total dose of local anesthetic administered to avoid exceeding the recommended top doses. In the first hour of surgery, the previous fast fluid deficit should be replaced and then administer adequate volume to obtain diuresis of 0.5 mL/kg/hour.

In our opinion, general anesthesia should be avoided and reserved for very select, complex cases or for patients who cannot tolerate or cooperate with conscious sedation [6]. The selection is indistinct and must be based on the physical conditions of the patient. In Lotus Med Group, we use isoflurane, sevoflurane, or desflurane and avoid or minimize the use of muscle relaxants. When the patient is extubated, special attention should be paid to avoid coughing and bowing that may facilitate bleeding in the surgical site.

Autologous fat grafting. Autologous fat grafting refers to the transfer of fat from one or more areas to other areas to improve body contouring. It is in vogue among plastic surgeons and their patients. It is a natural filler, available, and easy to obtain, which is usually reintegrated in the receptor sites, although it has an unpredictable percentage of resorption. The most frequent areas where fat is transferred include the hips, buttocks, breast, face, and hands. A typical grafting procedure is done in three phases: harvesting of adipose tissue from the donor area; processing of the lipoaspirate to eliminate cellular debris, acellular oil, and excess of infiltrated solution; and reinjection of the adipose tissue at the receptor site [67–69]. Lumbar approached subarachnoid anesthesia is the technique of choice when the fatty tissue to be extracted is below T4–T6, to be subsequently grafted to the buttocks, breast, and/or hips. We have observed that spinal anesthesia decreases bleeding at the donor site when compared to general anesthesia and facilitates rapid recovery, with less postoperative pain and home discharge on the same day without complications.

7. Postoperative pain control

Acute postoperative pain is an unresolved issue, including plastic surgery patients. Most plastic surgery procedures are accompanied by moderate/intense postoperative pain that can be disabling and prolong the hospital stay. The multiple neural ending injuries in liposuction and tummy tuck, even muscle elongations during breast implants, are just some examples that make it necessary to plan a rational analgesic scheme. The ideal analgesia should start from the pre-anesthetic phase using preemptive and preventing drugs. The combined use of opioids with NSAIDs is the cornerstone in the prevention and management of pain after plastic surgery. The controversy not clarified about the utility versus the negative effects of cyclooxygenase inhibitors has favored multiple investigations whose results allow the safe use of these drugs. Celecoxib 400 mg preoperatively followed by 200 mg every 12 hours reduces pain; total dose of opioids facilitates early recovery [70]. Parecoxib 40 mg i.v. every 12 hours is effective, and when methylprednisolone 125 mg intravenously is associated before surgery, it significantly reduces emesis [71]. This combination also reduces postoperative fatigue. The combination of tramadol with ketorolac is part of our routine, being able to replace acetaminophen with codeine. Mild pain can be treated with acetaminophen-codeine or sodium metamizole (dipyrone). Pregabalin and gabapentin may have a preventive analgesic effect. Sener et al. [72] found that in patients of septorhinoplasty lornoxicam (25 mg/day) has better tolerability and postoperative analgesia than dipyrone (5 mg/day) administered with a system of analgesia i.v. controlled by the patient. Gabapentinoids (gabapentin, pregabalin) and ketamine have additive or synergistic effects that decrease the doses of anesthetics in the transoperative and opioids in the immediate postoperative period.

Although the analgesic mechanism of esmolol (ultrashort-acting cardio-selective β1-adrenergic receptor antagonist) is not well known [73], some clinical studies have resulted in a decrease in propofol during the induction of general anesthesia, a reduction of general anesthetics during maintenance, and a reduced dose of transoperative opioids, as well as it reduces immediate postoperative pain [74–76]. Its use in rhinoplasty seems to reduce the dose of opioids in the intraoperative period and the intensity of immediate postoperative pain [77, 78].

Regional analgesia, as mentioned before, has a very important role: local anesthesia infiltrations and interfacial, paravertebral, intercostal, or epidural blocks.

8. Criteria for home discharge and home follow-up

Outpatient or short-stay plastic surgery patients should observe home discharge criteria that have been established for other types of surgery. These basic criteria establish the home discharge of patients in a safe manner and avoid readmissions due to complications.

Hemodynamic stability	**The return of vital signs to pre-anesthetic figures is mandatory**
Alertness	Patient awake, well oriented. Spinal anesthesia favors this state of alert which facilitates optimal home discharges
Permeable oral route	Tolerate the intake of liquids or solids without nausea or vomiting
Analgesia	Controlled postoperative pain (EVA <2/10) with oral analgesics. Subarachnoid anesthesia with adjuvants provides a prolonged period of analgesia that facilitates early home discharge and reduces the dose of analgesics. It is convenient to prescribe a combination of opioid and non-opioid analgesics according to the expected postoperative pain and the profile of each patient
Spontaneous micturition	This is a controversial requirement. Some centers consider it as mandatory to avoid readmissions by bladder balloon. In our practice we do not consider this requirement as indispensable, and the patient is informed of the remote possibility of difficulty urinating. We avoid the use of intrathecal morphine to reduce this risk
Ambulation	Complete regression of the motor block is convenient. The patient can try to walk when he/she has recovered the perianal sensitivity and can flex and extend the foot. In some cases, it is feasible to discharge without 100% recovery
Headache	Although the classic CPPD is presented as of the second post-block day, there are patients who can develop it in the immediate postoperative period. It is prudent to investigate it with the patient semi-seated or standing
Other	Absence of bleeding at the operative site, ensure company, stay and transport to patients who do not drive, establish possible means of communication such as telephone, FAX, email

Table 11. Criteria for home discharge.

Uncontrolled pain, nausea, vomiting, and urinary retention are examples of frequent readmission to the surgical unit or hospital. In some patients it is not necessary to meet 100% of these discharge criteria, but they should be warned of the natural evolution of the gradual disappearance of the side effects of anesthesia and facilitate telephone communication with the surgical unit, the surgeon, and the anesthesiologist. They require appropriate postanesthetic and postsurgical indications, transportation, and occasional professional company. Each ambulatory surgery unit/hospital must have its own discharge criteria, in accordance with the published guidelines and with its own characteristics and needs of their patients: from simple scales to more elaborate procedures such as the new Postoperative Quality Recovery Scale (PQRS) assessment that evaluates six areas: physiological, nociceptive, emotional, daily activities, cognition, and general patient perspective [79]. **Table 11** shows the usual discharge home criteria. The proper information on the patient evolution at the recovery house or patient home favors the prevention and the opportune diagnosis of complications [80].

9. Preventive methods and complications

Medical ethics and government regulations emphasize excellent care and safeguard the health needs of patients. The correct and sensitive communication of this carefulness is essential for a correct anesthesiological care. The lesions associated with anesthesia are a frequent cause of morbidity and litigation, so it is mandatory to identify the common factors associated with peri-anesthetic injuries and thus reduces possible demands. In anesthesia for plastic surgery, as in other surgical procedures, cardiopulmonary events are the most common errors or incidents that cause severe neurological damage or death. The keys to prevent legal action against the anesthesiologist are simple acts such as establishing an adequate relationship with the patient and his family from the pre-anesthetic period, appropriate pre-anesthetic evaluation, filling out the informed consent, always using the correct monitoring, performing the best anesthesia, and postanesthetic care [14].

The complications in plastic surgery are due to four general factors: (a) characteristics of the establishment where the procedure is performed, (b) type of surgery and surgeon, (c) physical condition of the patient, and (d) quality of anesthesiological care. The study by Clayman and Caffe [81] conducted in Florida, USA, with deceased patients who had been operated in office-based surgery facilities found 36 deaths in 5 years, 18 related to plastic surgery, 3 of which were seen by non-plastic surgeons, and 12 under general anesthesia, 10 of which were administered by anesthesiologists and 2 by nurse anesthetists. Seven of these cases died before discharge and 11 after apparent appropriate discharge. The deaths that occurred before patients were discharged from hospital were due to bronchospasm, deep sedation, one related to illicit drug use, and the other to fatty embolism. Of the 11 patients discharged, seven died due to possible thromboembolism. In the rest, the cause of death was not determined. Most of these deaths could be avoided with simple measures such as adequate trans-anesthetic surveillance, prophylaxis of DVT/PE, and optimal patient selection.

Deep vein thrombosis and pulmonary thromboembolism. These two entities are complications frequently related to plastic surgery (liposuction and tummy tuck). The frequency of PE is variable: circular abdominoplasty (3.4%), simple tummy tuck (0.35%), tummy tuck plus another plastic surgery procedure (0.79%), and abdominoplasty plus an intra-abdominal procedure (2.17%) [82, 83]. The plication of the rectus abdominis and the use of abdominal strips favor the increase of intra-abdominal pressure, decrease in venous flow, venous dilatation, and loss of normal biphasic venous flow at the popliteal level. The true impact of compression garment devices on DVT is still unknown [84], and pharmacological and mechanical protocols for thromboembolic prophylaxis in abdominoplasty seem to have similar results. This type of patients must be managed with a perioperative prophylactic scheme including graduated compression stockings, intermittent pneumatic compression tools, venous foot pumps, and drugs such as low molecular weight heparin or low-dose unfractionated heparin (20 mg of enoxaparin or equivalent daily for a week). Aspirin has been used successfully in major orthopedic surgery [85] and could have utility in plastic surgery with the risk of DVT/PE. The use of direct and indirect factor Xa inhibitions and thrombin inhibitors may be contraindicated since they induce greater postoperative bleeding [86, 87]. There is controversy about the risk of combining two or more plastic surgery procedures or other types (hysterectomy, colpoplasty, cholecystectomy). From anesthesia view, it is known that if there is longer operative time there are more possibilities of complications (bleeding, atelectasis, DVT, PE, alterations of the immune response, among others). The surgical literature is contradictory, and there are studies that favor combinations [83, 86, 87] and others that do not support this procedure [86].

Emesis. Postoperative and post-discharge nausea and vomiting remain the common and upsetting complications after plastic surgery. These symptoms interfere with the comfort of patients; they can have harmful effects on the results of surgery favoring bleeding, delaying discharge, and increasing costs [74]. There are several preventive schemes that have shown their effectiveness at low costs; the most usual combinations are dehydrobenzoperidol-dexamethasone and dexamethasone-ondansetron. The setrons (ondansetron, dolasetron, granisetron, tropisetron, and palonosetron) belong to a group of antiemetics with selective and potent antagonist action on the serotonin receptors, which also have an action on gastrointestinal motility and which lack antidopaminergic activity. Propofol 10 mg administered at the end of anesthesia has an antiemetic effect. Metoclopramide continues to be used, although its low effectiveness compared to other drugs and its side effects has decreased its use. The combination of transdermal scopolamine with intravenous ondansetron is another effective management option [87]. Brattwall and his group [88] found an antiemetic effect of smoking in breast augmentation. A prophylactic multimodal antiemetic regimen, suitable hydration, and opioid-sparing postoperative analgesia will decrease postsurgical emesis.

Chapter 7 of this book discusses the most frequent and unusual complications of anesthesia and plastic surgery.

10. Challenges

The challenges in anesthesia for plastic surgery patients are multiple since it is about people with perfectionist ideas that seek to improve their self-esteem through showing a better figure. This special personality makes them to search for a surgical medical team that guarantees their idealized success, which is based on information lacking scientific basis. On the other hand, the increasing sites offering plastic surgery has favored a demand not only for quality but also for more accessible prices. This nonmedical challenge is combined with the challenges of anesthesiological care in healthy patients, in apparently normal cases, and in people with systemic comorbidities. Each of these groups always requires a scrupulous comprehensive preoperative medical assessment and the development of a modifiable anesthetic plan. Another problem is the short and mediate term follow-up of these patients, since one way to improve our anesthesiological techniques is to study the evolution outside the operating room. The anesthesiologist rarely can see this type of outpatient or short-stay patient. So, it is prudent to establish a means of communication from the time of the pre-anesthetic visit to a long postanesthesia period. The Internet is by far the most viable way to determine what kind of evolution each of these patients have, especially the study of complications.

Patient-tourists represent a significant challenge very little studied in plastic surgery. They are people who have traveled for several hours or days, who come from other countries and who usually have not had a surgical or pre-anesthetic evaluation. They must be evaluated quickly and correctly to determine their viability to the procedures they want. It is common to see uncommon pathologies that do not contraindicate anesthesia, but can influence perioperative pharmacological management [2, 89].

11. Conclusions

Ambulatory and short-stay plastic surgery is growing logarithmically around the world. Anesthesiologists are more often subjected to the challenge of providing anesthesia to these patients, who on the other hand are scheduled every day for longer procedures and high risks that previously disqualified them for outpatient procedures. To favor an adequate outcome in this group of ambulatory patients—healthy and not so healthy, anesthesiologists should be oriented to the rational use of short and intermediate action drugs, with the goal of reducing morbidity and mortality. Techniques to prevent pain, nausea and vomiting, and early ambulation will be the most accepted procedures. The anesthetic techniques for outpatient surgery differ greatly from the procedures for short-stay patients, since the latter are scheduled to remain hospitalized for a minimum of 24 hours, unlike outpatient in which to prolong their stay beyond 5 pm can be considered as a failure in the anesthetic plan. A short recovery time after anesthesia is very important for the patient, his doctors, and the surgical unit.

Plastic surgery performed in ambulatory surgery units has some potential benefits such as ease of programming, reduced costs, and comfort for the patient and surgical staff. On the other hand, the inconveniences of ambulatory anesthesia should be considered, such as nausea and vomiting, uncontrolled postoperative pain, unplanned hospitalization, and, finally, occasional death. The latter is the most feared and should not happen.

Ambulatory cosmetic surgeries can potentially be managed with any anesthesiological technique. Although most anesthesiologists use general anesthesia for these procedures, regional anesthesia techniques have shown certain advantages such as better pain control, attenuation of the response to operative stress, preserving perioperative immune function, better preservation of oxygenation and lung residual functional capacity, improvement of visceral vascular flow, early recovery of postoperative ileus, and reduction of venous thrombotic disease and pulmonary embolism.

Acknowledgements

We thank the images of www.anestesia-dolor.org for allowing us to publish it.

Conflict of interest

None.

Author details

Víctor M. Whizar-Lugo[1*] and Ana C. Cárdenas-Maytorena[2]

*Address all correspondence to: vwhizar@anestesia-dolor.org

1 Lotus Med Group. Intensive Care Unit, Hospital General de Tijuana, ISESALUD, Tijuana, BC, México

2 Lotus Med Group, Tijuana, BC, Mexico

References

[1] https://www.plasticsurgery.org/documents/News/Statistics/2016/plastic-surgery-statistics-full-report-2016.pdf

[2] Nassab R, Hammett N, Nelson K, Kaur S, Greensill B, Dhital S, et al. Cosmetic tourism: Public opinion and analysis of information and content available on the internet. Aesthetic Surgery Journal. 2010;**30**:465-469. DOI: 10.1177/1090820X10374104

[3] Scott DL. Ambulatory anesthesia for cosmetic surgery. In: Steele SM, Nielsen KC, Klein SM, editors. Ambulatory Anesthesia and Perioperative Analgesia. New York: McGraw-Hill; 2005. pp. 311-322

[4] Ibarra P, Arango J, Bayter J, Castro J, Cortés J, Lascano M, et al. Consenso de la Sociedad Colombiana de Anestesiología y Reanimación, SCARE, y de la Sociedad Colombiana de Cirugía Plástica sobre las recomendaciones para el manejo de pacientes electivos de bajo riesgo. Revista Colombiana de Anestesiología. 2010;**37**:390-403

[5] Cárdenas-Camarena L, Andrés Gerardo LP, Durán H, Bayter-Marin JE. Strategies for reducing fatal complications in liposuction. Plastic and Reconstructive Surgery. Global Open. 2017;**5**(10):e1539. DOI: 10.1097/GOX.0000000000001539

[6] Whizar LV, Cisneros CR, Reyes AMA, Campos LJ. Anestesia para cirugía facial cosmética. Anesthesiology in Mexico. 2005;**17**:117-131

[7] Whizar LV, Cisneros CR, Reyes AMA, Ontiveros MP. Combined Lumbar Spinal-Epidural Anaesthesia (CLSEA) with Hyperbaric 0.75% Ropivacaine Plus Clonidine for Breast and Abdominal-Pelvic Plastic Surgery. An Open Trial. Paris, France: WCA; 2004. p. CD231

[8] Pitanguy I. Body-contouring surgery. Bulletin de l'Académie Nationale de Médecine. 2003;**187**:489-491

[9] Whizar-Lugo V, Cisneros-Corral R, Reyes-Aveleyra MA, Campos-León J, Domínguez J. Anesthesia for plastic surgery procedures in previously morbidly obese patients. Anesthesiology in Mexico. 2009;**21**:186-193

[10] Heller J, Gabbay JS, Ghadjar K, Jourabchi M, O'Hara C, Heller M, et al. Top-10 list of herbal and supplemental medicines used by cosmetic patients: What the plastic surgeon needs to know. Plastic and Reconstructive Surgery. 2006;**117**:436-445. DOI: 10.1097/01.prs.0000197217.46219.a7

[11] Caldera PS, Ayala CJL, Cortés BB. Herbolaria y anestesiología. Estudio en pacientes mexicanos sometidos a cirugía ambulatoria. Anesthesiology in Mexico. 2008;**20**:45-48

[12] Chin SH, Cristofaro J, Aston SJ. Perioperative management of antidepressants and herbal medications in elective plastic surgery. Plastic and Reconstructive Surgery. 2009;**123**:377-386. DOI: 10.1097/PRS.0b013e3181934892

[13] Ang-Lee MK, Moss J, Yuan CS. Herbal medicines and perioperative care. JAMA. 2001;**286**: 208-216

[14] Whizar-Lugo V. Prevención en anestesiología. Anesthesiology in Mexico. 2009;**21**:118-138

[15] Caplan RA, Posner KL. Informed consent in anesthesia liability: Evidence from the Closed Claims Project. ASA Newsletter. 1995;**59**:9-12

[16] Chrimes N, Marshall SD. The illusion of informed consent. Anaesthesia. 2018;**73**:9-14. DOI: 10.1111/anae.14002

[17] Andersen LP, Werner MU, Rosenberg J, Gögenur I. A systematic review of peri-operative melatonin. Anaesthesia. 2014;**69**(10):1163-1171. DOI: 10.1111/anae.12717

[18] Su X, Wang DX. Improve postoperative sleep: What can we do? Current Opinion in Anaesthesiology. 2018;**31**(1):83-88. DOI: 10.1097/ACO.0000000000000538

[19] Borazan H, Tuncer S, Yalcin N, Erol A, Otelcioglu S. Effects of preoperative oral melatonin medication on postoperative analgesia, sleep quality, and sedation in patients undergoing elective prostatectomy: A randomized clinical trial. Journal of Anesthesia. 2010;**24**(2): 155-160. DOI: 10.1007/s00540-010-0891-8

[20] Mistraletti G, Paroni R, Umbrello M, D'Amato L, Sabbatini G, Taverna M, et al. Melatonin pharmacological blood levels increase total antioxidant capacity in critically ill patients. International Journal of Molecular Sciences. 2017;**18**(4). DOI: 10.3390/ijms18040759

[21] Dewinter G, Staelens W, Veef E, Teunkens A, Van de Velde M, Rex S. Simplified algorithm for the prevention of postoperative nausea and vomiting: A before-and-after study. British Journal of Anaesthesia. 2018;**120**(1):156-163. DOI: 10.1016/j.bja.2017.08.003

[22] Practice guidelines for moderate procedural sedation and analgesia 2018: A report by the American Society of Anesthesiologists Task Force on moderate procedural sedation and analgesia, the American Association of Oral and Maxillofacial Surgeons, American College of Radiology, American Dental Association, American Society of Dentist Anesthesiologists, and Society of Interventional Radiology. Anesthesiology. 2018;**128**(3):437-479. DOI: 10.1097/ALN.0000000000002043

[23] Desai M. General inhalation anesthesia for cosmetic surgery. In: Friedberg BL, editor. Anesthesia in Cosmetic Surgery. New York: Cambridge University Press; 2007. pp. 155-169

[24] Brandom BW. Ambulatory surgery and malignant hyperthermia. Current Opinion in Anaesthesiology. 2009;**22**:744-747. DOI: 10.1097/ACO.0b013e328332a45b

[25] Friedberg BL. Propofol-ketamine technique: Dissociative anesthesia for office surgery (a 5-year review of 1,264 cases). Aesthetic Plastic Surgery. 1999;**23**:70-75. DOI: 10.1007/s002669900245

[26] Capdevila X, Dadure C. Perioperative management for one day hospital admission: Regional anesthesia is better than general anesthesia. Acta Anaesthesiologica Belgica. 2004;**55**(Suppl):33-36

[27] Whizar LV, Flores CJC, Campos LJ, Silva V. Spinal anaesthesia for ambulatory and short stay plastic surgery procedures. Chapter 3. In: Topics in Spinal Anaesthesia. Croatia: InTech Company; 2014. pp. 39-66. DOI: 10.5772/58407

[28] Whizar-Lugo VM, Cisneros-Corral R, Reyes-Aveleyra MA, Campos-León J, Shakhov A. Anestesia subaracnoidea en cirugía plástica ambulatoria. Anesthesiology in Mexico. 2008; **20**:23-33

[29] Rätsch G, Niebergall H, Hauenstein L, Reber A. Spinal anaesthesia in day-case surgery. Optimization of procedures. Anaesthesist. 2007;**56**:322-327. DOI: 10.1007/s00101-007-1141-9

[30] Korhonen AM. Use of spinal anaesthesia in day surgery. Current Opinion in Anaesthesiology. 2006;**19**:612-616. DOI: 10.1097/ACO.0b013e32801042c7

[31] Kallio H, Snäll EV, Suvanto SJ, Tuomas CA, Iivonen MK, Pokki JP, et al. Spinal hyperbaric ropivacaine-fentanyl for day-surgery. Regional Anesthesia and Pain Medicine. 2005;**30**:48-54

[32] Lennox PH, Chilvers C, Vaghadia H. Selective spinal anesthesia versus desflurane anesthesia in short duration outpatient gynecological laparoscopy: A pharmacoeconomic comparison. Anesthesia and Analgesia. 2002;**94**:565-568

[33] Chilvers CR, Goodwin A, Vaghadia H, Mitchell GW. Selective spinal anesthesia for outpatient laparoscopy. V: Pharmacoeconomic comparison vs. general anesthesia. Canadian Journal of Anaesthesia. 2001;**48**:279-283

[34] Carrada PS, Whizar LV, Pérez OA, Cabrera MN. Incidencia de cefalea postraquia en pacientes jóvenes. Estudio doble ciego, comparativo con Atraucan 26, Quincke 26 y Whitacre 27. Revista Mexicana de Anestesiología. 1997;**20**:3-10

[35] Whizar LV, Flores CJC, Preciado RS. Intrathecal clonidine as spinal anaesthesia adjuvant. Is there a magical dose? Chapter %. In: Topics in Spinal Anaesthesia. Croatia: InTech Company; 2014. pp. 97-121. DOI: 10.5772/58712

[36] Kuusniemi KS, Pihlajamäki KK, Pitkänen MT, Korkeila JE. Low-dose bupivacaine: A comparison of hypobaric and near isobaric solutions for arthroscopic surgery of the knee. Anaesthesia. 1999;**54**:540-543. DOI: 10.1046/j.1365-2044.1999.00855.x

[37] Gupta A, Axelsson K, Thorn SE, Matthiessen P, Larsson LG, Holmstrom B, et al. Low-dose bupivacaine plus fentanyl for spinal anesthesia during ambulatory inguinal herniorrhaphy: A comparison between 6 mg and 7.5 mg of bupivacaine. Acta Anaesthesiologica Scandinavica. 2003;**47**:13-16

[38] Whizar LV, Carrada PS, Cisneros CR, Cortes GC. Solar. Migración subaracnoidea del catéter o del anestésico durante anestesia epidural-espinal combinada. Informe de un caso. Revista Mexicana de Anestesiología. 1997;**20**:91-95

[39] Hafezi F, Naghibzadeh B, Nouhi AH, Salimi A, Naghibzadeh G, Mousavi SJ. Epidural anesthesia as a thromboembolic prophylaxis modality in plastic surgery. Aesthetic Surgery Journal. 2011;**31**(7):821-824. DOI: 10.1177/1090820X11417424

[40] Caplan RA, Ward RJ, Posner K, Cheney FW. Unexpected cardiac arrest during spinal anesthesia: A closed claims analysis of predisposing factors. Anesthesiology. 1988;**68**:5-11

[41] Eldor L, Weissman A, Fodor L, Carmi N, Ullmann Y. Breast augmentation under general anesthesia versus monitored anesthesia care: A retrospective comparative study. Annals of Plastic Surgery. 2008;**61**:243-246. DOI: 10.1097/SAP.0b013e31815bfe98

[42] Lai CS, Yip WH, Lin SD, Chou CK, Tseng CK. Continuous thoracic epidural anesthesia for breast augmentation. Annals of Plastic Surgery. 1996;**36**:113-116

[43] Blanco R, Fajardo M, Parras Maldonado T. Ultrasound description of Pecs II (modified Pecs I): A novel approach to breast surgery. Revista Española de Anestesiología y Reanimación. 2012;**59**(9):470-475. DOI: 10.1016/j.redar.2012.07.003

[44] Garg R, Bhan S, Vig S. Newer regional analgesia interventions (fascial plane blocks) for breast surgeries: Review of literature. Indian Journal of Anaesthesia. 2018;**62**(4):254-262. DOI: 10.4103/ija.IJA_46_18

[45] Fusco P, Scimia P, Marinangeli F, Pozone T, Petrucci E. The association between the ultrasound-guided Serratus Plane Block and PECS I Block can represent a valid alternative

to conventional anesthesia in breast surgery in a seriously ill patient. Minerva Anestesiologica. 2016;**82**(2):241-242

[46] Pacik PT, Nelson CE, Werner C. Pain control in augmentation mammoplasty using indwelling catheters in 687 consecutive patients: Data analysis. Aesthetic Surgery Journal. 2008;**28**:631-641. DOI: 10.1016/j.asj.2008.09.001

[47] Rawal N, Gupta A, Helsing M, Grell K, Allvin R. Pain relief following breast augmentation surgery: A comparison between incisional patient-controlled regional analgesia and traditional oral analgesia. European Journal of Anaesthesiology. 2006;**23**:1010-1017. DOI: 10.1017/S0265021506000883

[48] Heesen M, Klimek M, Rossaint R, Imberger G, Straube S. Paravertebral block and persistent postoperative pain after breast surgery: Meta-analysis and trial sequential analysis. Anaesthesia. 2016;**71**(12):1471-1481. DOI: 10.1111/anae.13649

[49] Lehnhardt M, Homann HH, Daigeler A, Hauser J, Palka P, Steinau HU. Major and lethal complications of liposuction: A review of 72 cases in Germany between 1998 and 2002. Plastic and Reconstructive Surgery. 2008;**121**:396-403. DOI: 10.1097/PRS.0b013e318170817a

[50] Klein JA. Tumescent technique for local anesthesia improves safety in large-volume liposuction. Plastic and Reconstructive Surgery. 1993;**92**:1085-1098

[51] Thomas M, Menon H, D'Silva J. Surgical complications of lipoplasty—Management and preventive strategies. Journal of Plastic, Reconstructive & Aesthetic Surgery. 2010;**63**: 1338-1343. DOI: 10.1016/j.bjps.2009.06.046

[52] Mysore V. Tumescent liposuction: Standard guidelines of care. Indian Journal of Dermatology, Venereology and Leprology. 2008;**74**(Suppl):S54-S60

[53] Klein JA. Tumescent technique for regional anesthesia permits lidocaine doses of 35 mg/kg for liposuction. The Journal of Dermatologic Surgery and Oncology. 1990;**16**:248-263

[54] Ostad A, Kageyama N, Moy RL. Tumescent anesthesia with a lidocaine dose of 55 mg/kg is safe for liposuction. Dermatologic Surgery. 1996;**22**:921-927

[55] Rosenberg PH, Veering BT, Urmey WF. Maximum recommended doses of local anesthetics: A multifactorial concept. Regional Anesthesia and Pain Medicine. 2004;**29**(6): 564-575

[56] Böni R. Safety of tumescent liposuction. Praxis (Bern 1994). 2007;**96**:1079-1082

[57] Platt MS, Kohler LJ, Ruiz R, Cohle SD, Ravichandran P. Deaths associated with liposuction: Case reports and review of the literature. Journal of Forensic Sciences. 2002;**47**:205-207

[58] Cantarelli J, Godoy MF. Safe limits for aspirate volume under wet liposuction. Obesity Surgery. 2009;**19**:1642-1645. DOI: 10.1007/s11695-009-9958-8

[59] Hanke W, Cox SE, Kuznets N, Coleman WP 3rd. Tumescent liposuction report performance measurement initiative: National survey results. Dermatologic Surgery. 2004;**30**: 967-978. DOI: 10.1111/j.1524-4725.2004.30300.x

[60] Trott SA, Beran SJ, Rohrich RJ, Kenkel JM, Adams WP Jr, Klein KW. Safety considerations and fluid resuscitation in liposuction: An analysis of 53 consecutive patients. Plastic and Reconstructive Surgery. 1998;**102**:2220-2229

[61] Hoyos A, Perez ME, Guarin DE, Montenegro A. A report of 736 high definition lipoabdominoplasties performed in conjunction with circumferential vaser liposuction. Plastic and Reconstructive Surgery. 2018. DOI: 10.1097/PRS.0000000000004705

[62] Hoyos AE, Perez ME, Castillo L. Dynamic definition mini-lipoabdominoplasty combining multilayer liposculpture, fat grafting, and muscular plication. Aesthetic Surgery Journal. 2013;**33**(4):545-560. DOI: 10.1177/1090820X13484493

[63] Matarasso A, Matarasso DM, Matarasso EJ. Abdominoplasty: Classic principles and technique. Clinics in Plastic Surgery. 2014;**41**(4):655-672. DOI: 10.1016/j.cps.2014.07.005

[64] Matarasso A, Smith DM. Combined breast surgery and abdominoplasty: Strategies for success. Plastic and Reconstructive Surgery. 2015;**135**(5):849e-860e. DOI: 10.1097/PRS.0000000000001238

[65] Deleuze A, Gentili ME, Bonnet F. Regional anaesthesia for head and neck surgery. Annales Françaises d'Anesthèsie et de Rèanimation. 2009;**28**:818-823. DOI: 10.1016/j.annfar.2009.07.072

[66] Friedberg BL. Propofol in office-based plastic surgery. Seminars in Plastic Surgery. 2007; **21**(2):129-132. DOI: 10.1055/s-2007-979214

[67] Simonacci F, Bertozzi N, Grieco MP, Grignaffini E, Raposio E. Procedure, applications, and outcomes of autologous fat grafting. Annals of Medicine and Surgery. 2017;**20**:49-60. DOI: 10.1016/j.amsu.2017.06.059

[68] Bellini E, Grieco MP, Raposio E. The science behind autologous fat grafting. Annals of Medicine and Surgery. 2017;**24**:65-73. DOI: 10.1016/j.amsu.2017.11.001

[69] Cárdenas-Camarena L, Durán H. Improvement of the gluteal contour: Modern concepts with systematized lipoinjection. Clinics in Plastic Surgery. 2018;**45**(2):237-247. DOI: 10.1016/j.cps.2017.12.005

[70] Sun T, Sacan O, White PF, Coleman J, Rohrich RJ, Kenkel JM. Perioperative versus postoperative celecoxib on patient outcomes after major plastic surgery procedures. Anesthesia and Analgesia. 2008;**106**:950-958

[71] Romundstad L, Breivik H, Roald H, Skolleborg K, Haugen T, Narum J, et al. Methylprednisolone reduces pain, emesis, and fatigue after breast augmentation surgery: A single-dose, randomized, parallel-group study with methylprednisolone 125 mg, parecoxib 40 mg, and placebo. Anesthesia and Analgesia. 2006;**102**:418-425

[72] Sener M, Yilmazer C, Yilmaz I, Caliskan E, Donmez A, Arslan G. Patient-controlled analgesia with lornoxicam vs. dipyrone for acute postoperative pain relief after septorhinoplasty: A prospective, randomized, double-blind, placebo-controlled study. European Journal of Anaesthesiology. 2008;**25**(3):177-182

[73] Ander F, Magnuson A, de Leon A, Ahlstrand R. Does the β-receptor antagonist esmolol have analgesic effects?: A randomised placebo-controlled cross-over study on healthy volunteers undergoing the cold pressor test. European Journal of Anaesthesiology. 2018; **35**(3):165-172. DOI: 10.1097/EJA.0000000000000711

[74] Gelineau AM, King MR, Ladha KS, Burns SM, Houle T, Anderson TA. Intraoperative esmolol as an adjunct for perioperative opioid and postoperative pain reduction: A systematic review, meta-analysis, and meta-regression. Anesthesia and Analgesia. 2018; **126**(3):1035-1049. DOI: 10.1213/ANE.0000000000002469

[75] Watts R, Thiruvenkatarajan V, Calvert M, Newcombe G, van Wijk RM. The effect of perioperative esmolol on early postoperative pain: A systematic review and meta-analysis. Journal of Anaesthesiology Clinical Pharmacology. 2017;**33**:28-39. DOI: 10.4103/0970-9185.202182

[76] Thiruvenkatarajan V, Watts R, Calvert M, Newcombe G, Van Wijk RM. The effect of esmolol compared to opioids on postoperative nausea and vomiting, postanesthesia care unit discharge time, and analgesia in noncardiac surgery: A meta-analysis. Journal of Anaesthesiology Clinical Pharmacology. 2017;**33**(2):172-180. DOI: 10.4103/0970-9185.209747

[77] Vahabi S, Rafieian Y, Abbas Zadeh A. The effects of intraoperative esmolol infusion on the postoperative pain and hemodynamic stability after rhinoplasty. Journal of Investigative Surgery. 2018;**31**(2):82-88. DOI: 10.1080/08941939.2016.1278288

[78] Celebi N, Cizmeci EA, Canbay O. Intraoperative esmolol infusion reduces postoperative analgesic consumption and anaesthetic use during septorhinoplasty: A randomized trial. Revista Brasileira de Anestesiologia. 2014;**64**(5):343-349. DOI: 10.1016/j.bjane.2013.10.015

[79] Stevens WG, Repta R, Pacella SJ, Tenenbaum MJ, Cohen R, Vath SD, et al. Safe and consistent outcomes of successfully combining breast surgery and abdominoplasty: An update. Aesthetic Surgery Journal. 2009;**29**:129-134. DOI: 10.1016/j.asj.2008.12.002

[80] De la Torre A, Rubial M. Anestesia en cirugía ambulatoria. Criterios de alta domiciliaria. Anales del Sistema Sanitario de Navarra. 1999;**22**(Supl 2):101-106

[81] Clayman MA, Caffee HH. Office surgery safety and the Florida moratoria. Annals of Plastic Surgery. 2006;**56**:78-88

[82] Hatef DA, Trussler AP, Kenkel JM. Procedural risk for venous thromboembolism in abdominal contouring surgery: A systematic review of the literature. Plastic and Reconstructive Surgery. 2010;**125**:352-362. DOI: 10.1097/PRS.0b013e3181c2a3b4

[83] Alderman AK, Collins ED, Streu R, Grotting JC, Sulkin AL, Neligan P, et al. Benchmarking outcomes in plastic surgery: National complication rates for abdominoplasty and breast augmentation. Plastic and Reconstructive Surgery. 2009;**124**:2127-2133. DOI: 10.1097/PRS.0b013e3181bf8378

[84] Clayman MA, Clayman ES, Seagle BM, Sadove R. The pathophysiology of venous thromboembolism: Implications with compression garments. Annals of Plastic Surgery. 2009;**62**: 468-472. DOI: 10.1097/SAP.0b013e31818cd08c

[85] Lippi G, Cervellin G. Aspirin for thromboprophylaxis in major orthopedic surgery: Old drug, new tricks? Acta Bio-Medica. 2018;**89**(1):31-33. DOI: 10.23750/abm.v89i1.7121

[86] Rangaswamy M. Minimising complications in abdominoplasty: An approach based on the root cause analysis and focused preventive steps. Indian Journal of Plastic Surgery. 2013;**46**:365-376

[87] Gan TJ, Sinha AC, Kovac AL, Jones RK, Cohen SA, Battikha JP, et al. A randomized, double-blind, multicenter trial comparing transdermal scopolamine plus ondansetron to ondansetron alone for the prevention of postoperative nausea and vomiting in the outpatient setting. Anesthesia and Analgesia. 2009;**108**:1498-1504

[88] Brattwall M, Warren Stomberg M, Rawal N, Segerdahl M, Houltz E, Jakobsson J. Postoperative impact of regular tobacco use, smoking or snuffing, a prospective multi-center study. Acta Anaesthesiologica Scandinavica. 2010;**54**:321-327

[89] Whizar-Lugo V, Flores-Carrillo JC, Campos-León J, Parra-Beltrán P, Azamar-Llamas D. Perioperative care of tourist-patients. Journal of Anesthesia & Critical Care: Open Access. 2015;**3**(6):00119. DOI: 10.15406/jaccoa.2015.03.00116

Chapter 2

Brain Monitored Propofol Ketamine for Elective Cosmetic Surgery

Barry L. Friedberg

Additional information is available at the end of the chapter

http://dx.doi.org/10.5772/intechopen.71442

Abstract

Brain monitored level of propofol hypnosis provides a numerically reproducible paradigm to block negative ketamine side effects. 50 mg IV ketamine 3 minutes prior to local anesthetic injection blocks virtually all midbrain NMDA receptors and is the basis for nonopioid preemptive analgesia. Opioid avoidance essentially eliminates postoperative nausea and vomiting (PONV) as well as the need for antiemetic agents. Over the past 20 years, no elective cosmetic surgical cases required hospital admission for either postoperative pain control or PONV.

Keywords: brain monitoring, BIS/EMG, propofol, ketamine, nonopioid preemptive analgesia (NOPA), PONV

1. Introduction

Elective cosmetic surgery *excludes* medically indicated procedures like postmastectomy breast reconstruction, burn and tendon repair that are the more properly included in the area of plastic surgery. As such, general anesthesia (GA) risks that may be acceptable for *medically indicated*, plastic surgery patients may not be acceptable for elective cosmetic surgery patients. Cosmetic surgery is "want to" surgery. Plastic surgery is "have to" surgery.

While all cosmetic surgery can be performed under local anesthesia only, most surgical candidates desire to not hear, feel or remember their procedures. Most surgeons prefer to concentrate on their surgery and not to have to speak with their patients during surgery. As such GA is commonly requested by many surgeons. Brain monitored propofol ketamine ("Goldilocks") anesthesia (not too much, not too little, but just right) bridges the patient care gap between surgery under local only and the more commonly performed GA. "Goldilocks" anesthesia

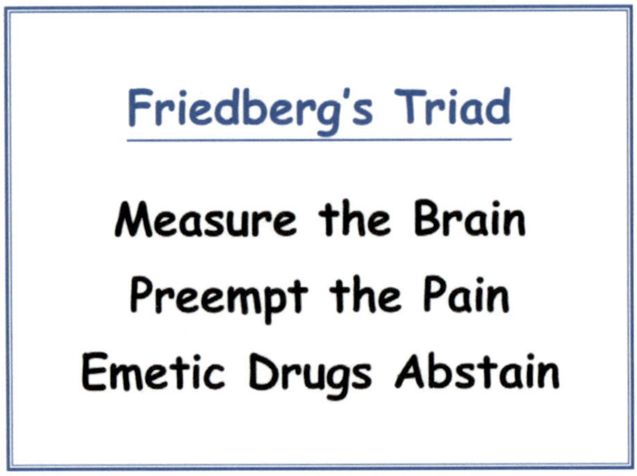

Figure 1. Friedberg's triad.

simulates GA conditions (nonverbal, predominantly immobile patients) while *trespassing the least* on patient physiology, satisfying both patient and surgeon desires. "Goldilocks" anesthesia is **numerically reproducible**. "Goldilocks" anesthesia embodies Friedberg's triad; i.e. Measure the brain, Preempt the pain, Emetic drugs abstain (**Figure 1**).

2. Direct cerebral cortical (brain) monitoring

> *When you can **MEASURE** what you are speaking about, and express it in **NUMBERS**, you know something about it; but when you cannot measure it, when you cannot express it in numbers, your knowledge is of a meager and unsatisfactory kind; it may be the beginning of knowledge, but you have scarcely, in your thoughts, advanced to the stage of **SCIENCE**.*
>
> *William Thompson, knighted Lord Kelvin Popular lectures and addresses 1891–1894.*

What was true for temperature measurement more than a century ago is also true for the direct measurement of patient's cortical response to anesthetics. Without such measurement, there can be no science. Without science, there can be no reproducibility across the broad, and often unpredictable yet well-recognized, spectrum of individual patient response to medications.

Brain weight does not vary with body weight (i.e. the brain weight of a 100-kg male is **NOT** twice that of a 50-kg female). Traditional anesthetic dosing based on body weight does not account for individual sensitivities to medications and is, therefore, frequently in error.

Further adding to the possibility of dosing error is the twentieth century practice of relying on heart rate (HR) and blood pressure (BP) changes to ascertain cortical drug response. **HR and BP changes primarily reflect brain stem response but are unreliable to accurately determine cortical response.** Prior to the ability to measure cortical response, the knowledge gap between brain stem and cortical response led to routine overmedication (to avoid under medication with awareness and recall).

Pain and consciousness are processed at higher cortical levels (**Figure 2**). Fifty percent of patients experiencing awareness with recall under anesthesia had no HR or BP changes with which to alert their anesthesiologist [1]. Preventing anesthesia awareness is the *least* important value of direct brain monitoring. No deaths have yet been reported from anesthesia awareness. However, one American overmedication death occurs daily! [2]. **Preventing over medication** is the major value of direct brain monitoring (**Figure 3**).

Complex mathematical modeling, i.e. pharmacodynamics (PD) and pharmacokinetics (PK), is based on body weight that may not accurately reflect individual cortical sensitivities. While currently unavailable in the US, target controlled infusion (TCI) only infers cortical response based on blood drug concentrations, again with possible error.

With the Federal Drug Administration (FDA) 1996 approval of the bispectral index™ (BIS) brain monitor, the promise of *direct measurement* of cortical hypnotic response to anesthetic drugs was made available to the anesthesia community. Competing cortical monitors have been introduced since 1996, but the BIS monitor remains the most well-validated brain monitor on the market to date.

Anesthesia may be defined as the sum of hypnosis plus analgesia (**Figure 4**). Implicit in "hypnosis" is amnesia for surgery and within "analgesia" is sufficient muscle relaxation to imbricate the rectus abdominis sheath for classical abdominoplasty. Measured hypnosis enables differentiation of cortical- versus spinal cord–originated patient movement. As opposed to cortically originating patient movement, spinal cord–originated patient movement is devoid of awareness with recall concerns. Knowledge of the origin of patient movement facilitates origin-appropriate treatment of patient movement, thus assuring adequate local anesthesia during sedation (**Table 1**).

As an index, the BIS scale is from 0 to 100. The lower the number, the deeper the level of hypnosis (**Table 2**). Although validated in over 3500 published papers, the promise of direct

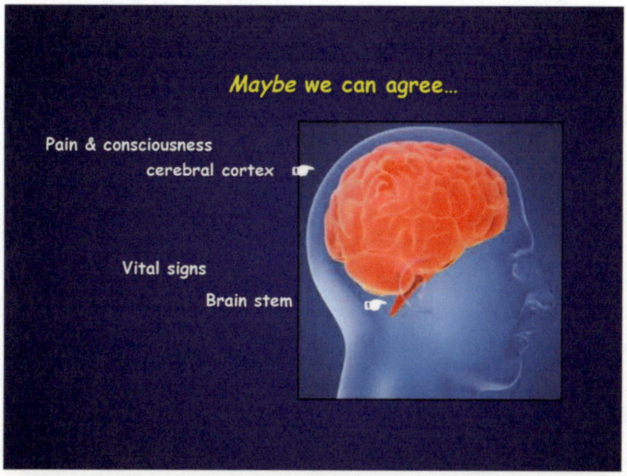

Figure 2. Cortex and brain stem.

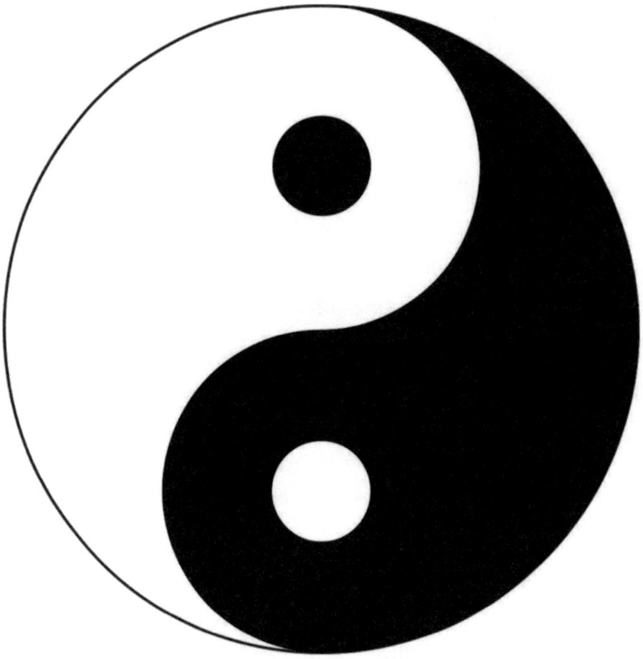

Figure 3. Hypnosis + analgesia = anesthesia.

brain monitoring has remained unrealized for several reasons. First, the BIS only measures response to hypnotic, not analgesic, drugs primarily acting of the cerebral cortex like propofol and inhalation agents like isoflurane, sevoflurane and desflurane. Drugs that act at lower brain centers are benzodiazepines (i.e. diazepam and midazolam), opioids (i.e. morphine, meperidine, hydromorphone, fentanyl, sufentanil, alfentanil, remifentanil), and N_2O. One cannot depend on reliable BIS cortical measurement from subcortically acting agents.

Second, the original factory default setting included only the BIS value and horizontally displayed BIS trend. BIS values are calculated by an algorithm that delays data by 15–30 s from real time. This delay puts the anesthesiologist in the unfavorable position of catching up to dynamically changing patient hypnotic requirements as opposed to having real-time information with which to formulate a response ahead of patient movement. BIS without EMG is *not useful* and is akin to trying to drive a car with only the rearview mirror information.

The electromyogram (EMG) is the electrical activity of the *frontalis* muscle between the eyebrows. This EMG is as real time and as instantaneous a signal as that of the EKG of the cardiac muscle. Unfortunately, the EMG was originally perceived as a "contaminant" of the BIS signal and not understood as a useful piece of information. *Prompt attention* to EMG spikes during sedation by increasing sedation to return the activity to baseline precludes "contamination" of the BIS value. Trending EMG spike activity enables the anesthesiologist to proactively respond to rapidly changing patient needs, providing a stable level of hypnosis throughout a case. BIS **with** EMG trending is very useful and is akin to driving a car looking through the forward-facing windshield.

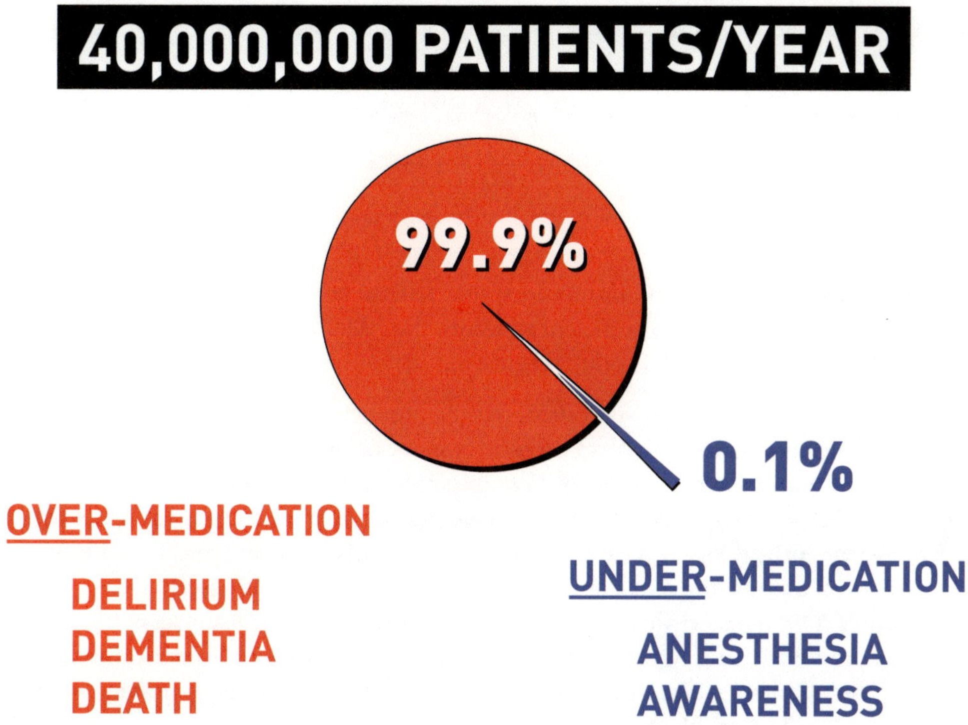

Figure 4. The value proposition of direct cortical monitoring.

BIS values	Hypnotic sedation/anesthesia levels
98–100	Awake
78–82	Minimal sedation
70–80	Moderate sedation
60–70	Deep sedation
45–60 + systemic analgesia	General anesthesia
<45	**OVERMEDICATED**

Table 1. BIS values and hypnotic sedation/anesthesia levels.

Anesthesiologists process information most consistently on the horizontal sweep as displayed in the EKG and SpO_2 trends. EMG is displayed on the original factory default, but only as a vertical column. Contained in the software of every free-standing BIS unit is the option to select EMG and save it to trend below the BIS trend on a horizontal sweep display. As of 2017, the factory default setting now displays both BIS and EMG trends. However, the lower EMG trend as pictured by the recent company literature is without important EMG spikes.

There are two vertical numerical scales on either side of the BIS monitor display (**Figure 5**). The left side scale (yellow) for the BIS is from 0 to 100. The right side scale (red) is from 30 to

Propofol titrated to 60 < BIS < 75 with baseline EMG indicated an asleep, amnestic patient.
A blanched surgical field does not equal adequate local analgesia.
Surgery below the clavicles with patient movement without EMG activity indicates more local analgesia in the immediate area of stimulation.

Table 2. The surgeon's golden rules for success with brain monitored propofol ketamine.

100 for the EMG. Spikes in EMG signify incipient patient arousal demanding an increase in propofol (or inhalational agent) sufficient to return the EMG to baseline (i.e. 0 on the top BIS scale and 30 on the bottom EMG scale). **(Figure 6)**.

In the pre-BIS era, anesthesiologists considered the absence of HR and BP changes with skin incision to define adequate depth of anesthesia. Nondissociative attempts at preemptive anesthesia have met with variable successes. Postoperative pain management continues to be an issue. HR and BP primarily reflect brain stem changes, while pain and consciousness are processed at higher cortical levels. Twenty-first century standard of care anesthesia monitoring demands cortical monitoring as a standard of care. It is an untenable assertion that 16 million of the 40 million (40%) American patients every year emerge from anesthesia with "brain fog" caused by a previously undiagnosed, underlying condition. Without numerically measuring the depth of sedation/anesthesia, discovering the role of routine overmedication in postoperative "brain fog" will be problematic [3].

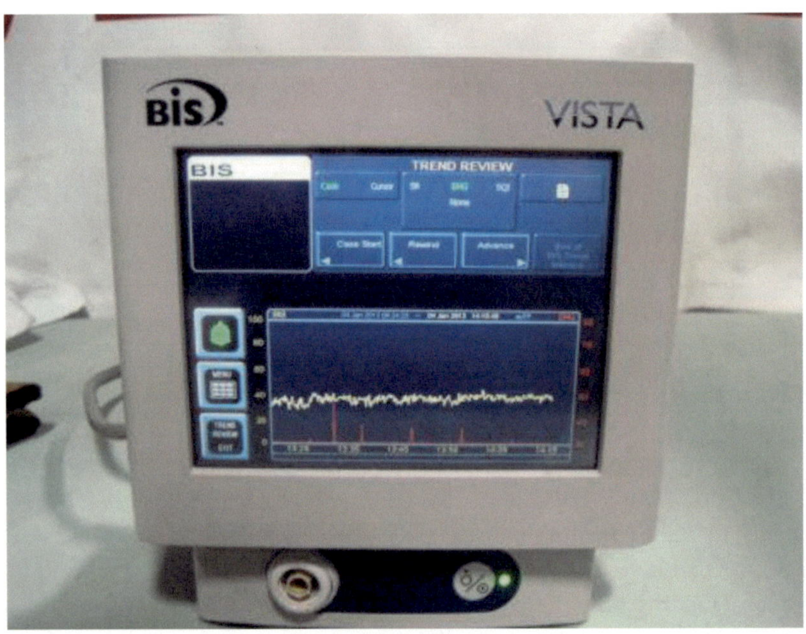

Figure 5. BIS VISTA monitor.

Once sedated, the brain cannot differentiate the signal from a well-intentioned surgeon's scalpel (or trocar) and the malevolent intentions of a mugger's knife. Success with preemptive analgesia makes it imperative to prevent the brain from receiving the noxious input from the violation of the integument's barrier to the outside world of danger. Although other pain receptors exist within the body, the most significant information to prevent the wind-up phenomenon and postoperative pain is that of skin incision.

The N-methyl, D-aspartate (NMDA) receptors in the midbrain are the final gatekeepers of noxious input to the cortex. Ketamine is a major NMDA antagonist (propofol has substantially less NMDA antagonism than ketamine). When the initial local anesthetic injection is performed (common to virtually all elective cosmetic surgeries), the **absence of an EMG spike** with multiple local anesthetic injections defines midbrain NMDA receptor saturation and creates nonopioid, preemptive analgesia.

Absent the ability to differentiate cortical- from spinal cord–originating movement during sedation forced anesthesiologists to treat every patient movement "as if" the patient might be awake and recall his or her surgery. All patient movement does not have the same significance. Like GA, "Goldilocks" anesthesia requires patients to be retrained on the operating table. Patient movement per se can be generated without cortical input, i.e. from spinal cord reflexes. A headless chicken still generates movement.

No spinal cord pathways exist to activate the facial *frontalis* muscle. During the case, patient movement without an EMG spike is an indication for additional local anesthesia in the immediate area of surgical stimulation. Only after two attempts of reinjection after the initial injection (three total injections) fails to eliminate patient movement should additional ketamine be given. Conversely, if patient movement is accompanied by an EMG spike, both additional local anesthesia **and** additional propofol should be administered. Additional local anesthetics should cause the patient movement to cease in the overwhelming majority of cases. Additional propofol must be administered in sufficient amounts to **return the EMG to baseline** to maintain the patient unconscious and amnestic.

It is not the absolute value (or spike) of any individual BIS reading that may determine recall. Rather, it is the area under the trend curve. Three to five minutes of a BIS >80 will more likely produce recall than less area under the curve. Restraint from the surgeon or operating room staff making loud, negative comments with patient movement deprives the unconscious patient subliminal input with which to process memories. One cannot control the emotional maturity of the personnel in the operating room. Many times, demonstrating to both the surgeon and his staff of an objective numerical measure of the patient's level of consciousness (i.e. BIS < 75 with baseline EMG) can calm otherwise overanxious personalities and preserve a peaceful operating room.

The use of EMG spike activity enables the differentiation between cortically generated patient movement and that originating from the spinal cord. Conducting a cosmetic surgery case in this fashion assures the patient receives critical adequate local anesthesia for the case and sets the stage for minimal postoperative pain management.

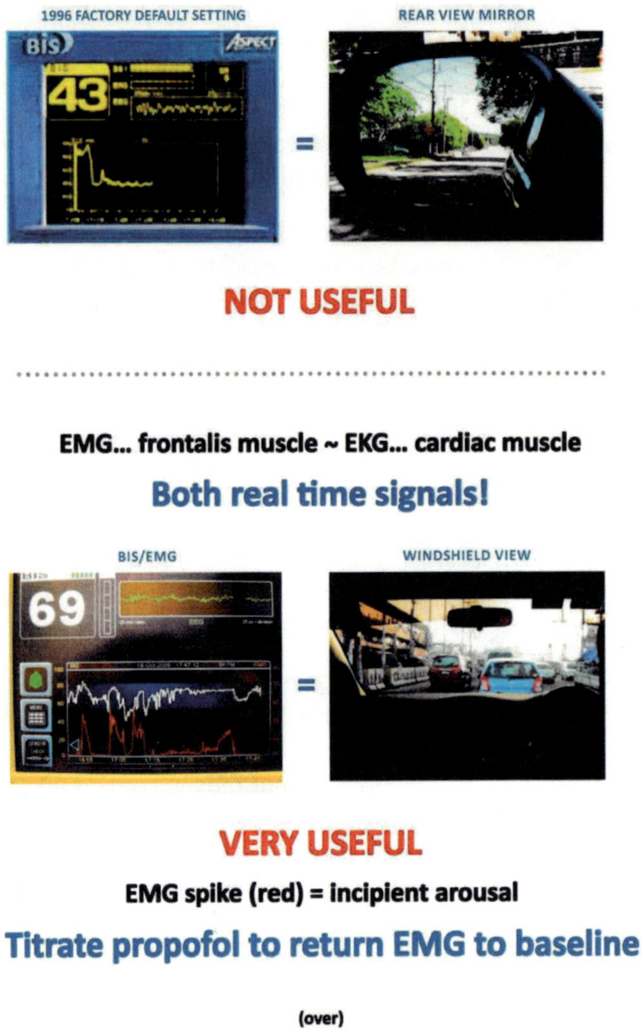

Figure 6. Why BIS is not commonly utilized.

Over the past two decades of experience in >4000 patients, the infrequent postoperative discomfort was readily managed with intravenous (IV) ketorolac 30–60 mg and/or oral acetaminophen 1000 mg. Rapid propofol emergence allowed patients who did request additional analgesia to safely swallow oral acetaminophen without aspiration risk. Higher acetaminophen blood levels are unquestionably achieved with the IV versus the oral preparation. However, since adequate pain relief was observed with the oral form, cost considerations precluded the use of IV acetaminophen. Very few patients required IV fentanyl (25–100 mcg) for pain management. The author's experience was entirely in the office-based setting. There were no postoperative hospitalizations for postoperative pain management during the period 1992–2017 in >6000 patients.

Prior to BIS/EMG monitoring, treating all movement left many patients overmedicated and unable to quickly emerge from anesthesia to go home or to a recovery center. Patient movement during sedation was generally regarded by the surgeon that the patient was "too light" and needed more sedation. Anesthesiologists often responded to the surgeon's demand with "needs more local." A circular argument ensued, physicians' feelings got bruised, but more importantly, the patient was ill-served, overmedicated, and often, with postoperative pain management issues.

The net effect of pre-BIS/EMG sedation attempts resulted in many surgeons encouraging (or even demanding) the abandonment of sedation in preference to GA with neuromuscular blocking agents. GA exposes the elective cosmetic surgery patient to the unnecessary risks of difficult intubation, failed intubation, misplaced endotracheal tube (ET), esophageal or endobronchial intubation, kinked or occluded ET, teeth damage, anesthesia machine mishaps (i.e. empty vaporizer, vaporizer filling error, reversed oxygen and nitrous oxide gases) and, very rarely, malignant hyperthermia (MH). No endotracheal intubations were required in the author's 25-year experience.

The advent of the use of the laryngeal mask airway (LMA) has greatly reduced or eliminated many ET issues. This author routinely places an armored (or flexible) LMA for rhinoplasty cases both to cover the glottic chink and using the inflatable cuff to prevent blood from entering the esophagus. For nonrhinoplasty cases, airway management is dependent upon patient response (**Table 3**).

The very small MH risk necessitates any GA facility stocking dantrolene, an expensive agent with a 3-year shelf life. Delays in treating MH are prompt recognition due to its rare occurrence and partly due to the difficulty of dissolving the treatment into solution to administer. A newer formulation of dantrolene (i.e. Ryanodex®) is easier to dissolve into solution for administration but may not be widely found.

Neither propofol nor ketamine is a triggering agent for MH. The early diagnosis of MH is most often made by unexplained tachycardia. Tachycardia is frequently observed following the injection of epinephrine containing local anesthesia at the beginning of the case. When the injection is temporally associated with the dissociative ketamine dose, some are more apt to believe the ketamine, not the epinephrine, was the source of the tachycardia. Often, in the performance of "Goldilocks" anesthesia, incremental propofol induction followed the ketamine, but the surgeon did not inject the local analgesia by as along as 10 minutes after the

Chin extended, head rotated to the side (initially to the right but sometimes better airway results turning to the left).
IV bag (not heated) under the shoulders (not the neck), increasing the force of extension on the genioglossus muscle.
#28 Fr latex (or latex free) lubricated nasal airway, often better tolerated than oral airways.
#4 LMA.
N.B. 50–60% of brain monitored PK cases/25 years have been performed without airway instrumentation. No endotracheal intubations required in 25 years, >6000 patients.

Table 3. Airway management flow chart (assumes incremental propofol induction).

ketamine administration. No tachycardia or hypertension was observed when ketamine was administered well prior to the lidocaine with epinephrine solution injection. Nontriggering "Goldilocks'" anesthesia also means surgical facilities need not stock dantrolene.

3. Propofol

Propofol is a 1,4-diisopropyl quinol with sedative-hypnotic properties. Because of its slight solubility in water, the drug is formulated as an emulsion for clinical use. It is highly lipophilic and distributes extensively in the body. The drug was introduced to the North American market in 1989 and has largely displaced both thiopental and methohexital for induction of general anesthesia and maintenance of sedation.

Propofol's rapid metabolism accounts for its short activity. It is also a potent antiemetic, especially in the absence of concomitant opioid administration. Only after much experience with the drug for sedation was the patients' clear head and happy affect after emergence was this quality appreciated by the author. Unfortunately, these qualities have also made propofol a drug of abuse within small numbers of the profession ("white rabbit") as well as by celebrities like Michael Jackson.

Propofol also results in inhibition of the N-methyl, D-aspartate (NMDA) subtype of glutamate receptor [4]. Lack of recall was observed in 95% of patients at BIS of 77 [5]. Propofol at 25–50 mcg/kg/min was sufficient to produce sedation to 60 < BIS < 75 with baseline EMG for many patients. However, as little as 2.5 mcg/kg/min and as much as 200 mcg/kg/min have been required to achieve the same numerically defined level of sedation at 60 < BIS < 75 with baseline EMG. This 20-year experience represents nearly a hundred-fold variation in propofol requirements. Incrementally inducing patients starting with 50 mcg/kg propofol miniboluses (*Watch YouTube Propofol induction with BIS monitor without instrumenting airway*) allows the anesthesiologist to identify outliers early in the case and enables all patients to receive "not too much, too little, but just the right amount" and not to hear, feel or remember their surgery. The expression "not too much, too little, but just the right amount" is the basis for using the shorthand expression "Goldilocks" anesthesia. Those unfamiliar with the Goldilocks story should watch YouTube Goldilocks and the Three Bears—Fairy Tales.

Textbook doses for propofol sedation do not discuss the value of incremental induction not only to identify outliers but also to dramatically minimize airway management and eliminate precipitous blood pressure drops. Incremental propofol induction more often maintains the airway patency by preserving muscle tone of the *temporalis, masseter, genioglossus* and *orbicularis oris*.

Propofol was introduced to North America in 1989 and quickly replaced both thiopental and methohexital as the preferred induction agent. As a proprietary agent, a 20 cc propofol bottle retailed around $12–15 USD, making a continuous infusion for surgery apparently prohibitive for multihour surgeries in a cost-conscious office-based cosmetic surgery suite.

After five years of performing propofol ketamine (PK) intravenous sedation using an average three 20 cc bottles of propofol per hour, the author's surgeons kept clamoring for a less expensive way to administer it, especially for 4–6 hours rhytidectomies with or without browlifts, platysmal plications or blepharoplasties. Five years of data on 1264 patients demonstrated no reduction in propofol requirements with either 2 or 4 mg preoperative midazolam as administered [6].

This same paper [6] also published the lowest postoperative nausea and vomiting (PONV) rate (0.6%) in the literature without antiemetic use in an Apfel-defined high-risk patient population, i.e. nonsmoking females with positive PONV and/or motion sickness histories, having emetogenic (cosmetic) surgery. Scrupulous opioid avoidance both during and after surgery has allowed this astounding PONV rate to go unchallenged to date.

Aspect Medical Systems (Aspect Medical Systems, a venture capital company, was purchased by Medtronic that has subsequently been acquired by Covidien) exhibited their bispectral index monitor™ (BIS) for measuring cortical effect at the 1997 International Anesthesia Research Society (IARS) annual meeting in San Francisco. The author was exhibiting his Society for Office Anesthesiologists (SOFA) at the same meeting and was initially exposed to the BIS monitor there. The BIS monitor appeared to offer more promise reducing propofol requirements than previous efforts with midazolam premedication [6]. Later work validated that promise [7, 8]. Entropy™ is another depth of anesthesia monitor but has not been validated in nearly as many clinical papers as BIS [9].

4. Ketamine

In the 1950s, postoperative pain was treated with morphine or meperidine, often undertreated for two reasons: (a) fear of producing opioid addiction and (b) problems of overtreatment, respiratory insufficiency or apnea and death. Naloxone was not introduced until 1971 and pulse oximetry became commercially available in 1983.

The researchers of the day postulated that, if another class of drugs could be developed that would ameliorate pain without respiratory depression, patients could be better treated for postoperative pain with neither under- nor overtreatment.

The first class of drugs explored was the phencyclidines. The parent compound, phencyclidine phosphate, was marketed as Serenyl® by Parke-Davis in 1958 but was quickly withdrawn from the market because of the high percentage of undesirable side effects, i.e. hallucinations, mania, delirium and disorientation. Later, phencyclidine phosphate, as a drug of abuse, became better known by the initials, PCP or "angel dust."

The researchers did not give up quickly on the phencyclidine class. They began experimenting with a modified PCP molecule, ketamine, which received FDA approval in humans in 1971. The drug, like its predecessor, was introduced as the "silver bullet," a complete, total intravenous agent, meaning no other agents were needed. Because it supported both respiration and blood pressure, ketamine quickly gained a reputation as a safe drug but one not good for adult patients. It did become popular in children's burn units, especially for the extremely painful dressing changes.

During the author's anesthesia residency at Stanford 1975–1977, he was introduced to administering ketamine in small doses (10–20 mg IV) prior to positioning elderly patients about to receive spinal anesthesia for surgery on femoral head or shaft fractures. Elderly patients were not particularly susceptible to ketamine-associated hallucinations or dysphorias. Veterinarians also adopted ketamine, quickly realizing that it was nearly impossible to kill an animal, even if the per body weight dose was more than twice the recommended amount. Also, the animals did not complain about hallucinations. While ketamine was a safe drug, two generations of human anesthesiologists have avoided its use in adult day surgery. Sometime during the mid-1970s, a Las Vegas plastic surgeon, Charles Vinnik, wearied listening to his patients cry out when he injected local anesthesia under his self-directed diazepam and meperidine IV sedation. Even though the patients had amnesia for the experience, the patients' cries were distressing to the OR staff. Vinnik asked his anesthesiologist if there was anything else he could use that would eliminate the distressing reactivity of the patients. Ketamine was suggested. Ketamine was first synthesized by Stevens in 1962 and first used in humans by Domino and Corssen in 1965. The drug was used in clinical practice barely 5 years when its use was suggested to Vinnik.

Through trial and error, Vinnik came upon his initial ketamine dose of 75 mg independent of body weight to prevent the patients from either moving or crying out after they were rendered sleepy from incremental doses of intravenous diazepam. Vinnik began with his test dose of 10 mg diazepam administered through an external jugular (to avoid venous thrombosis), followed by 5–10 mg increments to a total of 25–50 mg. Vinnik had his patients engage a 24-hour nurse to observe them after discharge to home. His cost-effective concept meant the cost of the recovery nurse did not come from him.

Although Vinnik published his diazepam-ketamine technique (i.e. **hypnosis first, then dissociation**) without the reported hallucinations or dysphorias, the 1981 paper appeared in the plastic surgery literature [10]. Vinnik's approach lay largely unnoticed in the anesthesia community until the author heard him speak in Newport Beach, CA, in December 1991, later visiting his office operating room in March 1992.

The author considered Vinnik's use of ketamine useful but doubted diazepam would be an optimal drug for day cases expected to return to home. Propofol was then considered as an alternative to diazepam for hallucination-blocking purpose. Searching the anesthesia literature to support this use of propofol turned up no useful information. March 26, 1992 was the beginning of this author's clinical trial of propofol followed by ketamine [11]. In the 1990s, ketamine became a drug of abuse, a "rave" drug and later lumped together with flunitrazepam and gamma hydroxybutyrate (GHB) as "date rape" drugs. Ketamine is also a drug of abuse. Heavy users can develop long-term bladder or urinary tract damage and incontinence.

Anesthesia trainees continue to be taught ketamine causes tachycardia, hypertension and hallucinations despite the knowledge that benzodiazepines [12] or propofol hypnosis blocks ketamine hallucinations [13]. In the pre-BIS era, loss of lid reflex and loss of verbal response defined adequate hallucination-blocking depth of propofol hypnosis. With real-time BIS/EMG monitoring, the level of hallucination-blocking propofol hypnosis is more numerically defined as $60 < BIS < 75$ with baseline EMG. Some believe the use of ketamine defeats the ability of the BIS monitor to accurately measure propofol. This study compared ketamine doses of 0.2–0.5 mcg/kg and concluded 0.5 mcg/kg would defeat the BIS [14]. An earlier publication using **50 mg ketamine, independent of body weight**, confirmed BIS' utility [15].

More controversial is the author's use of **50 mg ketamine *independent* of body weight**. Brain weight does not vary with body weight (i.e. the brain weight of a 100-kg male is not twice that of a 50-kg female). The midbrain is a very small portion of the total brain weight. The NMDA receptors are a small part of the very small midbrain. After observing the same immobility (or dissociative effect) in 100-kg males as in 50-kg females, body weight was not deemed a consideration for effective ketamine dose. With the addition of BIS/EMG monitoring, absence of EMG spike is considered numerically reproducible evidence of NMDA saturation and nonopioid, preemptive analgesia.

In many third world countries, ketamine infusions are still to be found as the drug was originally marketed. However, as propofol has become generic and very inexpensive, more anesthesia providers from third world countries have accessed the author's web site to obtain information with which to execute the PK paradigm.

Ketamine, ironically, is the perfect adjuvant drug (or the 'olive' in the propofol 'martini') not the complete and total intravenous agent its makers originally intended it to be, at least in the western world.

Brain monitored PK IV sedation is less expensive, safer and simpler and gives better outcomes (i.e. virtually no PONV [16] and minimal postoperative pain). With ability to stratify anesthesia outcomes by depth of anesthesia and the negative effects of routine anesthesia overmedication (i.e. BIS <45), studies have demonstrated more apparent negative effects from this practice [17–20]. Postoperative cognitive dysfunction (POCD) is the name for the pseudo-Alzheimer's type of confusion seen more often in elderly, rhytidectomy patients. Sometimes this lasts hours, days, weeks or months. Sometimes the effects are not transitory. Rapid emergence does not preclude intraoperative overmedication. Patients are left with the long-term consequences of their anesthesiologist's short-term care.

The brain monitored PK IV sedation technique also gives providers the ability to refrain from the nefarious practice of routinely overmedicating patients for fear of undermedicating them.

5. Putting brain monitored propofol ketamine ("Goldilocks") anesthesia into practice

Teaching the technique is simple. Teaching cooperation is not.

Daniel HS Lin, DO, Cosmetic surgeon

Along with the patient, many egos enter the operating room, not the least of which is that of the surgeon's. The surgeon's cooperation with local anesthesia is essential for success. The surgeon must also understand the need for *adequate* local anesthesia. **Surgeon perfection injecting local analgesia is not a requirement, only persistence.** Surgeons typically equate a blanched surgical field with adequate analgesia. Only with brain monitoring can the anesthesiologist hope to convince the surgeon that a blanched field only equals adequate vasoconstriction.

Prompt essentially PONV free and minimal pain recovery are the hallmarks of "Goldilocks" anesthesia. Once the surgeon observes how much better his patients do postoperatively, the need for his/her cooperation should become apparent. The office-based setting has a higher incentive for surgeon cooperation. Recovery space is limited and personnel are often multi-tasked compared with free-standing or hospital-attached day surgery center facilities. As superior and **numerically reproducible** as the "Goldilocks" anesthesia outcomes are, there are still surgeons reluctant to cooperate. Just as disappointing is the numbers of anesthesiologists who remain shackled to the outdated teachings that ketamine causes hallucinations, hypertension and tachycardia or are unwilling to reconsider using real-time BIS/EMG to titrate propofol.

The clinical pathway for brain monitored propofol ketamine ("Goldilocks") anesthesia is a simple straightforward three-drug technique: glycopyrrolate, propofol and ketamine. Induce hypnosis first, next dissociate, then inject local analgesia (**Table 4**). (Atropine may be substituted when glycopyrrolate is unavailable. Tachycardia will more commonly result than administering glycopyrrolate). Unexplained tachycardia, not temperature elevation, is the cardinal recognition sign for MH. Once the brain is protected with propofol incrementally titrated to loss of lid reflex/loss of verbal response or 60<BIS<75 with baseline EMG, the 50mg ketaamine by itself does not cause tachycardia or hypertension!

Prior to placing the BIS sensor on the forehead, the patient is advised **the number from their forehead allows them to "control" their anesthetic dose**. This control means that neither too much nor too little can be given. Then the patient is encouraged to touch the sensor pad to assure them their skin cannot be scarred even though the sensor application will be a little uncomfortable. A small discomfort for a great relief about anesthetic dosing is greatly appreciated by patients. Patients are additionally advised that 5% or one in 20 may have pleasant, colorful dreams.

The preoperative consultation includes disclosure of the dry mouth and the need to maintain eye lubrication with ointment. Patients are told to expect blurry vision upon awakening and

Glycopyrrolate 0.2 mg with 30 mg lidocaine IV
Propofol 50–100 mcg/kg^{-1} minibolus repeated to 60 < BIS < 75 with baseline EMG
Propofol infusion rate start 25 mcg/kg^{-1}/min^{-1}
Adjust infusion rate as needed to maintain 60 < BIS < 75 with baseline EMG
Ketamine 50 mg IV 3 minutes prior to local analgesia injection
Lidocaine 1 mg/lb^{-1} or 2 mg/kg^{-1} IV STAT for laryngospasm
Labetalol 10 mg iv for HR > 100–110. Avoid if patient asthmatic

Table 4. Clinical pathway.

that it is resolved when the ointment is wiped from their eyes. One patient in the author's 40-year career became panic-stricken upon emergence thinking something bad had happened to her eyes. Full disclosure to avoid repetition of this unfortunate patient's experience is strongly recommended.

Ketamine increases salivation. Glycopyrrolate causes less tachycardia and, for that reason, is chosen as an antisialagogue in preference to atropine. Because propofol can sometimes cause patient discomfort, lidocaine is added to the glycopyrrolate. The patient is advised to tell the anesthesiologist if there is additional aching during induction so that more lidocaine can be administered. Propofol ache is more common with distally placed IV.

Between 1992 and 1997, a 50-ml IV bag with 400 mg (40 ml) propofol was connected to a 60 drops/ml IV set (mini-drip, pedi-drip, micro-drip). The initial rate was set to the patient's heart rate and adjusted until **loss of lid reflex** and **loss of verbal response** were observed. This was a **qualitative** approach that was far more subjective and less reproducible. After the demand for the propofol numbers for publication, the author began using an infusion pump. A completely programmable, albeit more expensive, infusion pump is better than less expensive, commonly found pumps that only permit settings of 25, 50, 75 or 100 mcg/kg/min. The ability to deliver a separate bolus in addition to maintaining an infusion rate is also important. This **quantitative** approach along with BIS/EMG monitoring makes "Goldilocks" anesthesia numerically reproducible.

Set the pump to deliver propofol for 50 mcg/kg minibolus. Induce with miniboluses given in *one after another* until a decrease in the real-time frontalis muscle electromyogram (EMG) is observed (see YouTube Going under with Goldilocks anesthesia). The BIS value and trend line will display behind the EMG as it is based on algorithm-derived information that is delayed from real time by 15–30 s.

The induction goal is to observe whether or not 25 mcg/kg/min basal infusion rate is sufficient to maintain 60 < BIS < 75 with baseline EMG. Bolus with 50–100 mcg/kg to maintain BIS <75 and upwardly adjust the basal propofol rate to 35–50 mcg/kg/min to maintain that level PRIOR to administering ketamine. Most patients have been maintained at 60 < BIS < 75 with baseline EMG with propofol 25–50 mcg/kg/min. However, as little as 2.5 mcg/kg/min and as much as 200 mcg/kg/min propofol have also been observed by the author in his 20-year, >4000 patient clinical experience.

Avoid the textbook advice of 1–2 mg/kg propofol bolus for induction. A bolus will produce peak propofol levels in the brain quickly and just as quickly begin to redistribute, decreasing a protective level just as the ketamine arrives to the brain. The brain may then not be protected from ketamine side effects when that drug is administered. The value of the brain monitored, incremental induction is providing a **numerically reproducible, stable propofol brain level to prevent negative ketamine side effects** [13]. The very sensitive as well as the very resistant patient can be identified from the outset of the case rather than trying to understand a body weight–derived dose effect. Lastly, the incremental propofol induction preserves baseline blood pressure as well as the muscles that maintain a patent airway, *i.e. the temporalis, masseter, orbicularis* and *genioglossus*. Nevertheless, one must always be prepared with available bag mask ventilation and suction for the exceptional patient, no matter how often it will be unnecessary.

Only after the patient's propofol level has stabilized should the 50 mg ketamine, **independent of body weight**, be given, **3 minutes prior** to local analgesia injection. Any patient movement accompanied with an EMG spike during injection must be given more propofol to drive the EMG spike back to the baseline. As little as repeated 100 mcg/kg propofol boluses or as much as 200–400 mcg/kg propofol boluses may be required. An upward basal rate should be considered to maintain the patient's propofol level at 60 < BIS < 75 *with* baseline EMG.

The surgeon should inject as much of the proposed surgical field(s) with the initial ketamine dose whenever possible. Review of 1000 patient records demonstrated 80% were performed with one or two 50 mg ketamine doses. **Aggregate ketamine doses greater than 200 mg were associated with prolonged emergence.** Many surgeons are concerned that the lidocaine or epinephrine effect will not last if a lengthy procedure is contemplated. Long experience with Klein's ultradilute solution [21] has shown that concern is unwarranted even in 6-hour cases. Ketamine is to facilitate a painless injection of **'virgin' surgical fields** and is not necessary for reinjections when needed.

6. Laryngospasm

The traditional crowing sound of incompletely closed vocal cords is rarely seen with "Goldilocks" anesthesia. The type of laryngospasm is characterized by complete vocal cord closure. The only prodrome is a cough or a sneeze. The **traditional remedies** of anterior jaw thrust and positive pressure ventilation are **ineffective** in dealing with ketamine-associated laryngospasm. The author has consistently been successful treating this type of laryngospasm with IV lidocaine 1 mg/lb or 2 mg/kg given STAT whenever a cough or sneeze is observed.

Spontaneous ventilation preservation is a hallmark of successful "Goldilocks" anesthesia. The use of succinylcholine (SCh) will produce a patient with very painful postoperative muscle pains. SCh is not recommended as it is an MH trigger as opposed to nontriggering propofol or ketamine. Nondepolarizing rocuronium in small doses is a possibility but also defeats the value of spontaneous ventilation even with its short duration of action. Propofol elevates the lidocaine seizure threshold. The author has not observed lidocaine-induced seizures when treating laryngospasm with IV lidocaine. However, in *extremely* rare cases, severe bradycardia, even asystole, may be seen with multiple IV lidocaine injections. Preemptive lidocaine should be considered optional. Consider deepening propofol level after 2–3 lidocaine doses are required to break the laryngospasm.

7. Pitfalls to avoid

Anytime the words propofol and ketamine are used, readers too often think ketofol, the admixture of the two agents in the same syringe [22]. There are many permutations of the ideal ratio of propofol to ketamine. Mixing the two agents makes it very difficult, if not impossible, to differentiate when adequate hypnosis occurs as well as when midbrain NMDA receptor saturation occurs. "Goldilocks" anesthesia provides numerically reproducible propofol levels to define adequate hypnosis as well as the absence of EMG spikes with local anesthesia injection to define midbrain NMDA receptor saturation (**Table 5**).

Propofol ketamine is like the martini cocktail wherein the propofol is the 'vodka' and the ketamine is the 'olive.' Ketofol is when the propofol in mixed with the ketamine. These are two very different approaches that should never be confused with one another. **Do not mix propofol with ketamine.**

Propofol hypnosis is protective of ketamine hallucinations [13]. **Do not give ketamine before propofol hypnosis.** Bolus propofol induction will not provide a stable CNS propofol level to protect against ketamine hallucinations. Do not induce with 1–2 mg/kg propofol boluses.

Propofol at BIS < 75 with baseline EMG is a numerically reproducible protection against ketamine hallucinations. **Do not give ketamine if BIS > 75 or EMG is not at baseline.**

Adequate local analgesia is critical to minimizing or eliminating the need for postoperative opioid pain rescue. Do not fail to have the surgeon reinject the immediate area of dissection when patient movement occurs *without* EMG spike and BIS < 75. More propofol or ketamine is an inadequate response for patient movement at BIS < 75 with baseline EMG. Adding opioids instead of more local analgesia is not only inadequate to correctly deal with insufficient local analgesia but also increases the probability of PONV.

Aggregate ketamine doses >200 mg is associated with prolonged emergence. **Do not exceed 200 mg ketamine or give ketamine in the last 20 minutes** of the case or use ketamine in cases less than 20 minutes. Spontaneous ventilation is a prized safety feature of "Goldilocks" anesthesia. **Do not introduce an MH trigger like SCH to treat laryngospasm.** Because of the

Do not mix propofol and ketamine. Titrate separately to define goals of adequate hypnosis and midbrain NMDA saturation.
Do not give ketamine before propofol.
Do not bolus propofol for induction. Incrementally induce.
Do not give ketamine at BIS > 75.
Do not fail to provide adequate local analgesia.
Do not give opioids in lieu of adequate local analgesia.
Do not give ketamine in lieu of adequate local analgesia.
Do not exceed an aggregate ketamine dose >200 mg.
Do not give ketamine in the last 20 minutes of a case or for cases <20 minutes duration.
Do not paralyze instead of using lidocaine to break laryngospasm.
Do not use succinylcholine instead of lidocaine to treat laryngospasm.

Table 5. Pitfalls to avoid.

subsequent need to support ventilation, rocuronium is not preferred over IV lidocaine even though postoperative muscle pain will not result from its use.

8. Conclusion

While many anesthesiologists have observed "Goldilocks" anesthesia administered for classical abdominoplasty, cognitive dissonance often prevents believing what they have witnessed. It is not unusual for anesthesiologists to observe patients recover in a manner totally unlike that of GA or neuraxial block for them to believe that what they formerly believed was a major invasive surgery performed with a minimally invasive anesthetic approach.

When the surgeon is properly prepared for his role giving adequate local analgesia, the stage is set for outstanding, reproducible anesthesia outcomes for elective cosmetic surgery. The anesthesiologist needs to understand the real-time value of BIS/EMG monitoring and use it for the benefit of the conduct of the case. It may also be necessary to overcome outdated, unproductive teaching about negative ketamine side effects.

Cosmetic surgery patients endeavor to improve their level of happiness by altering their body image. Propofol is a happy affect drug that nicely complements the mental recovery of these patients.

Author details

Barry L. Friedberg

Address all correspondence to: drbarry@goldilocksfoundation.org

Goldilocks Anesthesia Foundation, Newport Beach, California, USA

References

[1] American Society of Anesthesiologists Task Force on Intraoperative Awareness. Practice advisory for intraoperative awareness and brain function monitoring: A report by the American Society of Anesthesiologists task force on intraoperative awareness. Anesthesiology. 2006;**104**:847-864

[2] Li G, Warner M, Lang BH, Huang L, Sun LS. Epidemiology of anesthesia-related mortality in the United States, 1999-2005. Anesthesiology. 2009;**110**:759-765

[3] Friedberg BL. The tree, the forest and standard of care. British Journal of Anesthesia. 2015;**115**:i114-i121. DOI: https://doi.org/10.1093/bja/aev211

[4] Vuka J, Sites E, Reefers M. Intravenous Anesthetics in Miller's Anesthesia. Canada: Elsevier Saunders; 2015. p. 826

[5] Glass PS, Bloom M, Kearse L, Rosow C, Sebel P, Manberg P. Bispectral analysis measures sedation and memory effects of propofol, midazolam, isoflurane, and alfentanil in healthy volunteers. Anesthesiology. 1997;**86**:836-847

[6] Friedberg BL. Propofol-ketamine technique, dissociative anesthesia for office surgery: A five-year review of 1,264 cases. Aesthetic Plastic Surgery. 1999;**23**:70-74

[7] Friedberg BL, Sigl JC. Bispectral (BIS) index monitoring decreases propofol usage in propofol-ketamine office based anesthesia. Anesthesia and Analgesia. 1999;**88**:S54

[8] Friedberg BL, Sigl JC. Clonidine premedication decreases propofol consumption during bispectral (BIS) index monitored propofol-ketamine technique for office based surgery. Dermatologic Surgery. 2000;**26**:848-852

[9] Hans P, Dewandre PY, Brichant JF, Bonhomme V. Comparative effects of ketamine on Bispectral Index and spectral entropy of the electroencephalogram under sevoflurane anaesthesia. British Journal of Anaesthesia. 2005;**94**:336-340

[10] Vinnik CA. An intravenous dissociation technique for outpatient plastic surgery: Tranquility in the office surgical facility. Plastic and Reconstructive Surgery. 1981;**67**: 199-205

[11] Friedberg BL. Propofol-ketamine technique. Aesthetic Plastic Surgery. 1993;**17**:297-300

[12] Reves JG, Glass PSA, Lubarsky DA, MD ME. Intravenous anesthetics in Miller's Anesthesia. Canada: Elsevier Saunders; 2010. p. p347

[13] Friedberg BL. Hypnotic doses of propofol block ketamine induced hallucinations. Plastic and Reconstructive Surgery. 1993;**91**:196

[14] Sengupta S, Ghosh S, Rudra A, Kumar P, Maitra G, et al. Effect of Ketamine on BISPECTRAL INDEX during propofol-fentanyl anesthesia: A randomized, controlled study. Middle East Journal of Anaesthesiology. 2011;**21**:391-395

[15] Friedberg BL. The effect of a dissociative dose of ketamine on the bispectral index (BIS) during propofol hypnosis. Journal of Clinical Anesthesia. 1999;**11**:4-7

[16] Friedberg BL. Avoiding emetogenic triggers in the first place is more effective than using antiemetics. Anesthesia and Analgesia. 2008;**106**:1921-1922

[17] Evered LA, Silbert BS, Scott DA, Maruff P, Ames D. Prevalence of dementia 7.5 years after coronary rrtery bypass graft surgery. Anesthesiology. 2016;**125**:62-71

[18] Chan MT, Cheng BC, Lee TM. BIS-guided anesthesia decreases postoperative delirium and cognitive decline. Journal of Neurosurgical Anesthesiology. 2013;**25**:33-42

[19] Radtke FM, Franck M, Lendner J, Krüger S, Wernecke KD, et al. Monitoring depth of anaesthesia in a randomized trial decreases the rate of postoperative delirium but not postoperative cognitive dysfunction. British Journal of Anaesthesia. 2013;**110**:98-105

[20] Leslie K, Myles PS, Forbes A, Chan MTV. The effect of bispectral index monitoring on long-term survival in the B-Aware trial. Anesthesia and Analgesia. 2010;**110**:816-822

[21] Klein JA. Anesthetic formulation of tumescent solutions. Dermatologic Clinics. 1999: 751-759

[22] Andolfatto G, Abu-Laban RB, Zed PJ, Staniforth SM, Stackhouse S, et al. Ketamine-propofol combination (ketofol) versus propofol alone for emergency department procedural sedation and analgesia: A randomized double-blind trial. Annals of Emergency Medicine. 2017;**59**:504-512

Chapter 3

Pediatric Anesthesia for Patients with Cleft Lip and Palate

Alyssa Brzenski, Ofelia Ham-Mancilla,
Silvia Peña-Olvera, Amanda Gosman and
Alicia Sigler

Additional information is available at the end of the chapter

http://dx.doi.org/10.5772/intechopen.74926

Abstract

Cleft lip and palate are the most common craniofacial deformities in the United States of America and México. Their aesthetic and functional implications influence the lifestyle of the patient: social relationships, school and working performances, self-esteem and health. Surgical repair of the cleft lip is around the third to sixth month of age and the palate repair is when the patient is between six and eighteen months old. There are other surgical repairs during childhood and ideally all of them should be performed by an experienced surgeon teaming up with a pediatric anesthesiologist following the gold standards in cleft care, in a setting where the safety of the patient is paramount.

Keywords: cleft lip, cleft palate, anesthesia

1. Introduction

When anesthetic procedures are performed in cleft patients, there are multiple considerations that have to be taken into account: the actual lip and palate deformities that could lead to a difficult intubation, airway malformations and reactions to the procedure that could lead to laryngospasm or bronchospasm, other malformations or diseases that could alter the prognosis during and after the surgery, the surgical procedure itself that could lead to bleeding or airway obstruction due to swelling, the intubation, the administration of anesthetic medications, the ventilation and use of other medications such as muscle relaxants, pain killers, etcetera, that could alter the homeostasis of the body, and other factors surrounding the anesthetic procedure like the equipment used, the monitoring applied, the site where the surgical act is taking place, the experience of surgeons, anesthesiologists and nurses in charge of cleft care, the availability of a blood bank and an ICU in case of an adverse event. When all of these factors are well controlled and overseen by an experienced team, the risk for an adverse outcome is significantly reduced. This is why there has been an international consensus for guidelines that will lead the cleft team to successful surgical and anesthetic performances. If the team is visiting a foreign country, they must follow the same gold standards of care contained within these guidelines and work within their scope of practice. If the medical setting that they are visiting lacks the equipment, medications and supplies needed for them to perform at their best, then they should bring the equipment, medications and supplies with them.

2. General considerations

Cleft lip (CL) and cleft palate (CP) are one of the most common congenital anomalies found in the United States and the most common craniofacial anomaly seen by plastic surgeons. Nearly one in five hundred live births will result in a child affected by cleft CL and/or CP. The Center for Disease Control estimates that 2650 babies are born with CP and 4440 babies are born with CL with or without a CP annually [1]. In developing countries, such as México, CL and CP is the most common congenital malformation requiring surgical treatment and its incidence is 1:800 to 1000 live births. Of these, 33% have CL. 64% CL and CP. 2% only present a CP and 1%, rare craniofacial clefts. On average, there are 9.6 new cases per day and 3521 cases per year [2].

In the United States, children with CL and CP are primarily cared for in cleft centers with multidisciplinary teams. Teams consisting of otolaryngologists, plastic surgeons, oral surgeons, speech therapists, occupational therapists, dentists and orthodontists work together to ensure optimal timing and care of these patients. Anesthesiologists also integrate into these teams when surgical procedures are required. Studies from the United Kingdom suggest that children who are cared for by these multidisciplinary teams have improved long-term outcomes with improved feeding, speech, and esthetics [3–7]. For many families, the diagnosis of a cleft occurs during the prenatal period. Prenatal counseling may be the first interaction with the cleft team, facilitating a long relationship with multiple specialists to establish expectations regarding the long-term possibilities for children with CP or CL and CP. There are approximately 139,000 Mexicans who have CL and CP. It is a very important public health problem due to the medical, psychological and social impact to the patients and their family. The causes are multifactorial and can be environmental, genetic or a combination [8].

Infants with CL and CP can have difficulty generating oral suction which can make breast feeding and bottle feeding a challenge. Many infants with CL and CP struggle with feeding and may require special bottles, nipples or education to achieve adequate weight gain. Children without access to support services may endure nutritional consequences, which if not taken care of at an early age, can deteriorate or affect growth and development [2, 9].

The goals for surgical repair of CP and CL repair are to reconstruct the affected area, leading to improved feeding, speech, and function of the nasal airway. CL repair in the United States typically occurs first within 2 to 3 months of age with CP repair occurring between 9 and 12 months [10]. The time between birth and this initial repair allows for a thorough work up of other co-morbidities and evaluation of any underlying syndromes. In the majority of children with a cleft there are no other associate syndromes or malformations. However, 20–30% of patients will have some underlying syndrome or systemic abnormalities requiring evaluation and potentially treatment prior to repair of the cleft [11]. Isolated CP has the greatest incidence of associate abnormalities while isolated CL is most likely to be an isolated feature. Thus, a thorough pre-operative evaluation by the cleft team is essential prior to surgical repair.

At least 275 different syndromes [12] have been associated with CL and CP. There are a variety of co-morbidities associated with these syndromes. However, cardiac and airway abnormalities represent the primary concerns of the anesthesia teams prior to repair of cleft abnormalities. Syndromes such as Pierre Robin Sequence, Treacher Collins, Goldenhar Syndrome and 22q deletion, are associated with mandibular hypoplasia, potentially making airway management and repair difficult. Cardiac abnormalities are the most frequent associate co-morbidity in children with clefts [13]. Tetralogy of Fallot, atrial septal defect and ventricular septal defect represent the most common congenital heart disease seen in this patient population. A thorough physical exam and imaging with cardiac echocardiogram should be performed for these children. Cardiac abnormalities should be optimized and potentially repaired prior to repair of the cleft itself. Optimization of other co-morbidities, such as airway anomalies, renal dysfunction, nutrition and additional medical issues, should also be a top priority in the months following birth. Children with CP are prone to middle ear effusions and recurrent otitis media. The dysfunction of the palate muscles impairs regulation of the Eustachian tubes, which may increase the risk of upper respiratory infections.

Patients with CP have an increased risk of gastroesophageal reflux and pulmonary aspiration which may contribute to airway reactivity. Speech impairment also occurs due to the abnormal anatomy of the CP musculature and speech development is further hindered in patients with hypoacusia [12]. In México, the multidisciplinary approach is a must in almost all 53 cleft clinics located throughout the country and the role of the anesthesiologist is vital as well as the pediatrician, cardiologist, geneticist, nutritionist, pneumologist, gastroenterologist and all other specialists that may be involved in the preoperative assessment for the patient. Once the patient has undergone the lip and/or palate surgeries, the multidisciplinary cleft team involving the surgeon, orthodontist, speech therapist, otorhinolaryngologist, audiologist and psychologist become very active in providing their services to improve the physical appearance and the functional activity regarding speech, hearing, feeding, and socialization and self-esteem of the patient [14].

3. Consideration of anesthesia management

During surgical repair, a general anesthetic is required to allow for optimal surgical conditions. Control of ventilation through endotracheal intubation is necessary. Given the abnormalities of the face, concern may exist regarding the difficulty of mask ventilation and endotracheal intubation. Both ease of ventilation and intubation might have significant effects on the management of the induction of anesthesia as well as the equipment that should be present prior to induction of general anesthesia. Unlike the adult population, there are not any objective exam criteria that can help identify a difficult airway. Young children will not participate in the normal airway exam. A difficult airway, defined as a difficult laryngoscopy, intubation or mask ventilation, is less common in pediatric patients [15–20]. However, young age (less than 1 year of age) and craniofacial abnormalities increase the risk of a difficult airway [15].

Although there are not set criteria that is useful to identify a child with a CP who will be a difficult laryngoscopy, examination for retrognathia should occur in each child. Viewing the face from the side is an easy way to identify retrognathia. If retrognathia is present, a potentially difficult intubation should be anticipated, and additional precautions should be undertaken. In the United States, a laryngeal mask airway, video laryngoscope and a fiber optic bronchoscope are tools that could be used to aid with a difficult intubation. If providing surgical care in a resource limited location these tools may not be available. An honest, but thorough evaluation of the facility's capabilities should be performed to ensure that the primary goal of doing no harm to the patient is followed.

Pre-operative history should also focus on determining if the infant has an upper respiratory infection (URI). Patients with a URI are at increased risk for perioperative respiratory events such as bronchospasm, laryngospasms, desaturations, breath holding and postintubation croup [21]. Presence of copious sputum and secretions, nasal congestion, recent URI (less than 2 weeks), and history of reactive airway disease increased the risk of perioperative adverse respiratory events [22]. Patients with CL and/or CP with a recent URI are at an increased risk of perioperative respiratory events compared to children without CL and/or CP who have had a recent URI. To minimize the risk of perioperative respiratory events, it is recommended that surgery be postponed for 4–6 weeks after the URI has resolved and that an experienced pediatric anesthesiologist performs the anesthetic [19]. Despite these perioperative events, in the experienced hands of a pediatric anesthesiologist there is not a risk for substantial morbidity or mortality in these patients. Nonetheless, if these symptoms are present it is prudent to postpone surgery for repair of the CL or CP until the child is no longer ill. Gunawardana and Arteau-Gauthier et al. [23, 24] studied risk factors for difficult laryngoscopy in children with CP. These children did not have any identified syndrome. 5–7% of patients in these studies had difficult laryngoscopy, a higher incidence than in other pediatric patients. Large or bilateral clefts, micrognathia and age less than 6 months were associated with increased incidence of difficult laryngoscopy. Large and bilateral clefts can be difficult because the blade of the laryngoscope can fall into the cleft. Should this occur, one can pack the cleft with gauze to improve the laryngoscopy. No patients in these studies were associated with difficult mask ventilation. Since mask ventilation is not difficult in most of these patients, an inhaled induction with volatile anesthetic with control of ventilation is appropriate in most of these patients in experienced hands.

The preanesthetic assessment is very important and should contain the patient's information: age, height and weight and its main goals are:

a) To obtain the medical and surgical background of the patient:

- Family background of anesthetic problems
- Perinatal background such as pregnancy evolution, kind of delivery, complications during delivery, need of special care after birth, prolonged hospitalization [9].

- Non-pathologic background related with nutritional state and development
- Review of systems: pulmonary abnormalities including recent respiratory infections, craniofacial deformities that will make airway and respiratory management more difficult [8], cardiac abnormalities and their treatment and cardiovascular evaluation required latest respiratory infection due to the high incidence of fistula formation or palate wound dehiscence [8], or increasing the incidence of complications of the anesthetic procedure (23%). It has been recommended a period of 4 to 6 weeks between the relief of respiratory infection and the surgical and anesthetic event to avoid such complications [25–26]. Another important issue is allergies to medications, food and toys. Kind of malformations the patient has and other anesthetic procedures in the past and the patient's reactions to them.
- Complete physical examination, including the possibility of difficult venous access and airway.
- Lab work: complete blood count, prothrombin time, partial thrombin time, bleeding and coagulation times, and any other studies for cardiovascular assessment such as EKG, chest X-rays or echocardiogram [25].

b) Evaluate the anesthetic risk and decide on the anesthetic technique to be used.

c) Inform the parents about the anesthetic technique to be used and the possibility of adverse events as well as the amount of time the patient needs to be NPO before the surgery depending on the age of the patient: 2 hours of clear liquids in all ages, to age less than 6 months 4 hours for maternal milk, and 6 hours for non-maternal milk. For patients 6 to 36 months old; 6 hours to solid food and non-maternal milk including formula [26, 14].

d) Preoperative medications: intranasal dexmedetomidine is great for patients older than 6 months because it diminishes secretions that are produced by crying. It must be administered and be continuously monitored in any setting. Midazolam PO is used to treat separation anxiety before taking the children into the operating room.

No matter the setting where the cleft surgery is going to take place, the anesthetic procedure must have the basic monitoring like continuous evaluation of electrocardiography, noninvasive blood pressure, arterial oxygen saturation, temperature, end-tidal carbon dioxide, with capnography. The objective is to obtain a safe management of the patient and to minimize the complications [9, 27]. When the surgical outreach trips for clefts in children occur in a general hospital not a pediatric hospital, it is important to provide that institution with the appropriate monitors and equipment for the adequate management and safety for the patient.

There is no standard anesthetic that has been shown to be superior in the care of children for repair of CL and CP. Typically, CL are repaired at 2–3 months of age to improve feeding and repair the muscular of the mouth. CP is repaired between 9 and 12 months of age. The goal is to optimize speech development. However, earlier repair could increase the likelihood of midface hypoplasia in the future. No premedication is required for children of these ages undergoing CL and CP repair. At this stage in life, separation anxiety is not yet a major concern. Most children present for surgery from home and have no established intravenous access. Most anesthesiologists utilize an inhalational induction with volatile anesthesia. If a difficult airway is anticipated, then this induction may be changed. The induction stage is the one with the most risk of adverse events. The main adverse event reported in the literature at the Instituto Nacional de Pediatría in Mexico City is laryngospasm which was noted in 77% of the cases [28]. Once intravenous access is obtained intubation with a RAE (Ring, Adiar and Elwyn) endotracheal tube is used. The pre-formed bend in this endotracheal tube lies on the chin, optimizing the surgical exposure for the surgeon. For a CP repair a throat pack may be used and a Digman retractor is typically placed to further improve surgical visualization. Care must be taken to ensure that the endotracheal tube is not moved when these devices are placed, as endobronchial intubation or inadvertent extubation can occur. In addition, the Digman retractor can compress the endotracheal tube when initially raised. Communication with the surgeons is important to ensure optimal oxygenation and ventilation continues throughout the surgical repair. Multiple anesthesia techniques can be used for the children undergoing CL or CP repair. In the United States, use of a volatile anesthetic with or without opioids or regional anesthesia [29–31] is commonly used. Anesthesia with propofol-remifentanil can also be used with similar anesthetic results [30].

There is an important incidence of adverse events during this stage such as accidental extubation and occlusion of the endotracheal tube by surgical instruments or malposition of the patient. It's also important to mention the laryngospasm and bronchospasm during the palate repair. Hypothermia in patients of two months to two years of age is directly proportional to the length of the surgery and the temperature of the surgical room [27]. In the Instituto Nacional de Pediatría, hypothermia was a frequent concern and it is critical to keep the surgical room at an adequate temperature to avoid other adverse events that could alter the behavior or stability of the patient during the moment of the extubation. To avoid the adverse events such as laryngospasm and bronchospasm it is important to set criteria for the best moment of extubation.

4. Perioperative and postsurgery analgesia

Pain control during the entire perioperative procedure is especially important in CL and palate surgeries. Multi-modal pain therapy with narcotic, non-narcotic and regional anesthesia can help ensure optimal pain control. In the United States, the surgeon will typically inject local anesthetic and epinephrine prior to the repair of both CL as well as CP. The main goal of this injection is to provide vasoconstriction in surgical field. However, when local anesthetic is utilized the patient will benefit from some additional pain control. The duration of which is dependent on the type of local anesthetic used. Opioids can be used intraoperatively to smooth the hemodynamic response to surgical pain. Some anesthesiologists in the United States are increasingly using the short acting narcotic remifentanil. Remifentanil is potent and quick acting, but is metabolized quickly allowing its effects to dissipate quickly. Remifentanil can also be used to facilitate a smooth emergence and extubation in these patients. However, remifentanil may not be available in all facilities throughout the world, making it difficult to utilize in resource limited locations.

Regional anesthesia can provide excellent analgesia in children undergoing surgical repair of CL. The infraorbital nerve provides sensory innervation to the skin on the unilateral skin and mucous membranes from the upper lip through the check and to the lower eyelid. Sensory innervation for the nasal alae is also provided (**Figure 1**). Blockade of the infraorbital nerve should provide pain relief for most of the tissue affected by a CL repair. A 2016 Cochrane Review of infraorbital nerve blocks during CL repair demonstrated that bilateral infraorbital nerve blocks result in lower opioid consumption during the surgical procedure as well as lower pain scores in the Post-Anesthesia Care Unite (PACU) [32]. The pain relief was superior to fentanyl [33], placebo [34], and local infiltration [35]. Nicodemus et al. [36] demonstrated that pain relief lasted 19 hours when a mixture of bupivacaine with epinephrine was used for the block. Infraorbital nerve blocks can be easily placed via two approaches; intraoral or extra-oral. The intraoral approach directs a 25 g needle in the mouth and until the gingiva-labial fold near the canine toward the infraorbital notch. The infraorbital nerve emerges from the infra-orbital foramen below the eye which is easily palpated in most patients. Care must be taken to avoid advancing the needle past the foramen into the eye in neonates and infants. Given the small size of these patients, the toxic dose of local anesthesia should be calculated when the surgeon also utilizes local anesthetic with epinephrine for vasoconstriction in the surgical field. Typically, only 0.5–1 mL of local anesthetic is utilized.

The sensory innervation of the palate is more complex than the lip, requiring blockade of the greater palatine, lesser palatine and the nasopalatine. Each of these nerves is branches of the maxillary division of the trigeminal nerve. The suprazygomatic approach to maxillary nerve blockade allows a single injection to provide improved pain control for CP repair [37–38]. Overall, pain was better controlled, and fewer narcotics were required for the first 48 hours following

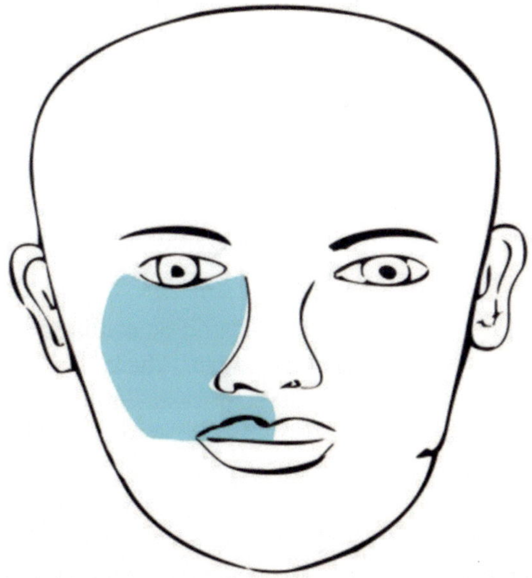

Figure 1. Sensory innervation of the infraorbital nerve.

surgical repair. Unfortunately, suprazygomatic maxillary nerve block is not frequently used due to lack of familiarity by most anesthesiologists in the United States currently. However, unlike infraorbital nerve blocks the nerve block alone is not sufficient to provide adequate analgesia. Typically, narcotics are used in the United States to supplement the residual discomfort.

Multi-modal pain management incorporates the use of non-narcotic medications. Acetaminophen, non-steroidal anti-inflammatory medications and the alpha-2 agonists, like dexmedetomidine, are commonly used in pediatric patients to reduce the total amount of opioids required following surgical procedures, and to reduce the side effects of opioids such as respiratory depression. In infants undergoing primary CP repair acetaminophen is effective in reducing pain scores and overall opioid consumption [39], with intravenous acetaminophen providing the lowest pain scores and lowest opioid consumption compared to placebo and oral administration. Rectal acetaminophen historically has been used given its ease of administration. However, overall opioid consumption is not decreased when rectal acetaminophen is used; suggesting other routes of administration might be preferred [40]. Alpha-2 agonists, such as dexmedetomidine, and ketamine given intraoperatively can also decrease postoperative pain [41].

5. Postoperative care

Postoperatively, there is not a concern for respiratory compromise with CL repair. CP repair differs as obstruction is possible following extubation. The surgical repair itself reduces the size of the airway and excessive sedation from anesthesia and opioids can cause the tongue to lose muscle tone causing obstruction. If the Digman retractor is up for long periods of time, the tongue itself can have some swelling. Obstruction is problematic as blind placement of an oral airway can result in disruption of the fresh surgical repair. Therefore, a plan should be formulated intraoperatively to avoid obstruction in the postoperative period. Dexamethasone is frequently given early during the surgical repair to reduce any swelling. A tongue stich or nasal trumpets can also be placed by the surgeon following CP repair to relieve obstruction should it result. These techniques are not uniformly used by cleft teams in the United States [42] and there is no increase in reintubation rates when tongue stitch is avoided [43], but it is our practice to place a tongue stitch on all our CP patients. The tongue stitch remains in place while the patient is in the PACU, but is removed before transfer to a medical floor for monitoring overnight.

During the postoperative stage, the main care is based on continuous monitoring the supplementary oxygen depending on the needs of the patient. The bleeding assessment is the proper management of pain and the start of oral intake of clear liquids before allowing the patient to be discharged. It is important to establish which patients are candidates for ambulatory management, which ones have a higher risk to present adverse events like bronchospasm, laryngospasm, desaturation and respiratory difficulty. High risk patients with palate repair could end up having to stay in the hospital or intensive care unit longer than expected and this should be a consideration [28]. It's recommended that the stay at the PACU is 1 hour at least [26]. In the Instituto Nacional de Pediatría in Mexico City, the management of pain after surgery is based on paracetamol at 15 mg/kg or an AINE like ketorolac at 1 mg/kg, and other

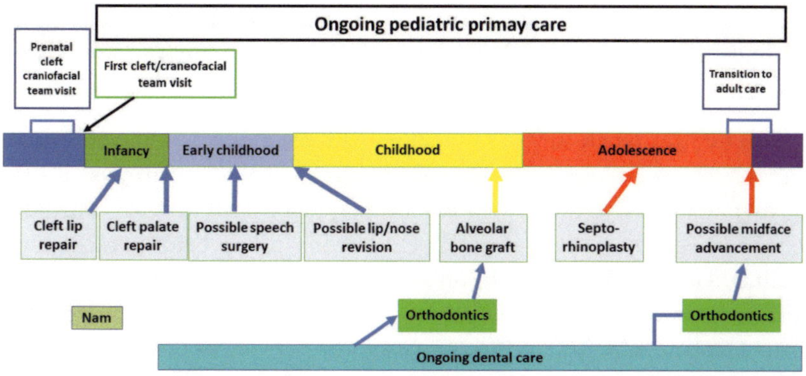

Figure 2. Edited from Lewis CW, Jacob LS, Lehmann CU, AAP SECTION ON ORAL HEALTH. The primary care pediatrician and the care of children with cleft lip and/or cleft palate [44].

options such as a combination of both, or paracetamol with an opioid such as tramadol, or AINE with an opioid. During the surgical outreach trips for clefts, at the surgical setting, there should always be a postanesthetic care unit well equipped to monitor and observe the pediatric patients. The availability of an intensive care unit and a pediatric ventilator should be part of the criteria for any site where one of these trips will take place.

Following the primary repair of CL and CP, children with CP with or without CL have multiple future treatments and potential additional surgical interventions (**Figure 2**).

After multiple surgical procedures, children can be anxious about future procedures. Any past stressful procedure may create lasting difficulty for the future perioperative period. The anesthesiologist should assess for anxiety and create a plan that eases the fears of the patient. In addition, anesthesiologists should be aware of past procedures and what was done. This is especially important following a pharyngoplasty. Nasal intubation following pharyngoplasty can tear or disrupt the past surgical repair. All attempts at nasal intubation should be avoided if possible.

6. The international team of cleft lip and palate

Internationally, there is a need for surgical teams to help aid in surgical repairs of CL and CP. A full discussion of the techniques of establishing sites for these surgical services is beyond the scope of this chapter. However, it is important for the anesthesiologists to recognize differences occur when surgical teams go to other countries. When resources are limited, the choices one makes may differ from the choices made in one's home country. Similarly, a different environment may affect outcomes [45]. Before proceeding with any medical procedures, it is helpful to understand local culture and medical practices. For example, in the United States it is very common that patients receive opioid medications for recovery on the hospital medical floor following surgery. In some countries, the infrastructure and the comfort with postoperative narcotics is not present. Thus, an adapted anesthetic plan should be implemented to ensure that the ultimate goal of adequate pain relief is met with non-narcotic medications. In these countries reliance in nerve blocks and other non-opioid pain medication becomes valuable (**Table 1**).

The most important idea when surgically treating patients in other countries is to remember to *"first do no harm."* The pre-operative evaluation becomes vital to ensuring safety in these kids. It is unlikely that an extensive cardiac evaluation may have been done. A murmur on exam or a history consistent with heart failure warrants further workup before proceeding to surgery. Similarly, a difficult airway should not be underestimated when in a resource limited location. If a potential difficult airway is identified, with known risk factors such as retrognathia, young age and a syndrome associated with a difficult airway, an assessment of resources is important. A plan should be made prior to proceeding in case extubation is not possible following the procedure. Finally, a history and physical should thoroughly inquire about the possibility of a current or recent upper respiratory infection. If risk factors for perioperative respiratory complications from the upper respiratory infection are identified, surgical repairs should be postponed.

In general, once appropriate surgical patients are identified, anesthetic care is similar regardless of the location. The medications available and local customs for postoperative care will help shape the anesthetic designed and the plan for postoperative care.

All reconstructive and craniofacial surgeons that oversee cleft care should treat any patient abroad as if they are at their usual surgical facility at home; always following the quality guidelines for their best performance and safety for the patients. There are different protocols for cleft care all over the world, but the visiting surgeon should adapt to the local multidisciplinary team in charge and ensure that there will be the proper follow up for the patients. A complete documentation should be the rule for the entire team working in the operating room. This will simplify preoperative assessment in the future and enable the team to properly evaluate current and future issues that could lead to any adverse outcome and will help

Syndromes associate with CL and CP	Common features
Pierre Robin Sequence	Micrognathia, glossoptosis
Treacher Collins syndrome	Micrognathia, ear defects, congenital heart disease
Goldenhar's syndrome	Unilateral mandibular hypoplasia, unilateral ear deformity
Down syndrome	Macroglossia, atlantoaxial instability, congenital heart disease
Fetal alcohol syndrome	Congenital heart disease, developmental delay
22q deletion syndrome	Congenital heart disease, hypocalcemia, thymic hypoplasia
Klippel-Feil syndrome	Fusion of the cervical spine, renal disorders
Stickler syndrome	Connective tissue disorder, glaucoma and cataracts, hearing loss, joint hypermobility

Table 1. Shows some syndromes associated with CL and/ or CP and common characteristics.

improve the quality of care provided. All facilities should meet the basic standards to care for all patients, if these standards are not met by the facility, the visiting team is required to bring with them the supplies and equipment necessary to meet these basic standards such as:

1. Electrical power that is dependable and continuous.
2. Working modern anesthesia machines.
3. Dependable oxygen supply.
4. Full-functioning monitoring for each patient in the operating rooms.
5. Working suction should be present at each operating room table and in the recovery area.
6. Basic laboratory and radiology services should be immediately available.
7. Blood banking.

Every team should include a surgeon who is familiar with the planned procedures, preferably a board certified surgeon, a board certified anesthesiologist experienced in the care for children undergoing same or similar procedures, who should be supervising no more than two procedures at any given time, certified nurse anesthetists with experience in the care of children undergoing the same or similar procedures, a board certified pediatrician, operating room, recovery area and ward nurses experienced in the care of children.

The visiting team should always bring the airway equipment including appropriate laryngoscopes and blades, laryngeal mask airways, self-inflating bag-valve-mask in all care areas, emergency cricothyroidotomy kit and fiber-optic bronchoscope. Emergency medications, emergency vascular access kits, defibrillator, portable pulse oximetry, Stat laboratory and portable oxygen supply must be included among the supplies and equipment needed during cleft surgical outreach trip [46].

7. Conclusions

Anesthesia in cleft patients should be performed in a setting with the proper equipment, medications and supplies to provide the safest procedure by experienced anesthesiologists since these patients have high risk for respiratory complications such as difficult intubation, laryngospasm, bronchospasm, or if they have had an upper respiratory infection within the month preceding the surgery, then they may suffer complications like pneumonia or bronchopneumonia. If any other complication may arise from the surgical or anesthetic procedure, the anesthesiologist should be able to diagnose it and manage it and the patient should be transferred to a post anesthetic care unit or intensive care unit, depending on the severity of the complication. Favorable outcomes are directly related to carefully selecting the patient that will undergo cleft surgery, anesthesiologists properly trained to manage this kind of cases and having all the human and material resources to provide the best care during and after the surgical procedure.

Conflict of interest

None of the authors have any conflict of interest.

Author details

Alyssa Brzenski[1], Ofelia Ham-Mancilla[2], Silvia Peña-Olvera[2], Amanda Gosman[3] and Alicia Sigler[4]*

*Address all correspondence to: aliciasiglerplasticsurgeon@gmail.com

1 University of California San Diego, San Diego, CA, USA

2 Instituto Nacional de Pediatría, Ciudad de México

3 UC San Diego School of Medicine, University of California San Diego, San Diego, CA, USA

4 Clínica Ambulatoria Shriners, Tijuana, Baja California, México

References

[1] Parker SE, Mai CT, Canfield MA, Rickard R, Wang Y, Meyer RE, Anderson P, Mason CA, Collins JS, Kirby RS, Correa A. National Birth Defects Prevention Network. Updated national birth prevalence estimates for selected birth defects in the United States, 2004-2006. Birth Defects Research. Part A, Clinical and Molecular Teratology. 2010;**88**(12): 1008-1016. DOI: 10.1002/bdra.20735

[2] Polaiah KP, Madhavi KN, Sivaiah T. A study of airway complications among the patients of cleft lip and cleft palate during intraoperative and postoperative period at government general hospital, Guntur. Journal of Evolution of Medical and Dental Sciences. 2015;**4**(9):1488-1492

[3] Al-Ghatam R, Jones TE, Ireland AJ, Atack NE, Chawla O, et al. Structural outcomes in the cleft care UK study. Part 2: Dento-facial outcomes. Orthodontics & Craniofacial Research. 2015;**18**(Suppl 2):14-24. DOI: 10.1111/ocr.12109

[4] Ness AR, Wills AK, Waylen A, Al-Ghatam R, Jones TE, et al. Centralization of cleft care in the UK. Part 6: A tale of two studies. Orthodontics & Craniofacial Research. 2015; **18**(Suppl 2):56-62. DOI: 10.1111/ocr.12111

[5] Persson M, Sandy JR, Waylen A, Wills AK, Al-Ghatam R, et al. A cross-sectional survey of 5-year-old children with non-syndromic unilateral cleft lip and palate: The cleft care UK study. Part 1: Background and methodology. Orthodontics & Craniofacial Research. 2015;**18**(Suppl 2):1-13. DOI: 10.1111/ocr.12104

[6] Sell D, Mildinhall S, Albery L, Wills AK, Sandy JR, Ness AR. The cleft care UK study. Part 4: Perceptual speech outcomes. Orthodontics & Craniofacial Research. 2015;**18**(Suppl 2): 36-46. DOI: 10.1111/ocr.12112

[7] Smallridge J, Hall AJ, Chorbachi R, Parfect V, Persson M. Functional outcomes in the cleft care UK study--part 3: Oral health and audiology. Orthodontics & Craniofacial Research. 2015;**18**(Suppl 2):25-35. DOI: 10.1111/ocr.12110

[8] Adenekan AT, Faponle AF, Fadekemi Oginni FO. Perioperative adverse airway events in cleft lip and palate repair. Southern African Journal of Anaesthesia and Analgesia. 2011;**17**(6):370-373. DOI: 10.1080/22201173.2011.10872808

[9] Gómez-García R, Lara-Navarro R. Incidencia de labio y paladar hendido en México: 2003-2006. Revista ADM. 2008;**45**(6):309-313

[10] Waylen A, Ness AR, Wills AK, Persson M, Rumsey N, Sandy JR. Cleft care UK study. Part 5: Child psychosocial outcomes and satisfaction with cleft services. Orthodontics & Craniofacial Research. 2015;**18**(Suppl 2):47-55. DOI: 10.1111/ocr.12113

[11] Dixon MJ, Marazita ML, Beaty TH, Murray JC. Cleft lip and palate: Understanding genetic and environmental influences. Nature Reviews. Genetics. 2011;**12**(3):167-178. DOI: 10.1038/nrg2933

[12] Leslie EJ, Marazita ML. Genetics of cleft lip and cleft palate. American Journal of Medical Genetics. Part C, Seminars in Medical Genetics. 2013;**163C**(4):246-258. DOI: 10.1002/ajmg.c.31381

[13] Wyse RK, Mars M, Al-Mahdawi S, Russell-Eggitt IM, Blake KD. Congenital heart anomalies in patients with clefts of the lip and/or palate. The Cleft Palate Journal. 1990; **27**(3):258-264

[14] López-Muñoz AC, Busto-Aguirreurreta N, Braulio T. Guías de ayuno preoperatorio: Actualización. Revista Española de Anestesiología y Reanimación. 2015;**62**(3):145-156. DOI: 10.1016/j.redar.2014.09.006

[15] Heinrich S, Birkholz T, Ihmsen H, Irouschek A, Ackermann A, Schmidt J. Incidence and predictors of difficult laryngoscopy in 11,219 pediatric anesthesia procedures. Paediatric Anaesthesia. 2012;**22**(8):729-736. DOI: 10.1111/j.1460-9592.2012.03813.x

[16] Lee A, Fan LT, Gin T, Karmakar MK, Ngan Kee WD. A systematic review (meta-analysis) of the accuracy of the Mallampati tests to predict the difficult airway. Anesthesia and Analgesia. 2006;**102**(6):1867-1878. DOI: 10.1213/01.ane.0000217211.12232.55

[17] Shiga T, Wajima Z, Inoue T, Sakamoto A. Predicting difficult intubation in apparently normal patients: A meta-analysis of bedside screening test performance. Anesthesiology. 2005;**103**(2):429-437

[18] Alarcón-Almanza JM. Labio y paladar hendido. Rev Mex Anestesiol. 2010;**33**(S1):S76-S78

[19] El-Ganzouri AR, McCarthy RJ, Tuman KJ, Tanck EN, Ivankovich AD. Preoperative airway assessment: Predictive value of a multivariate risk index. Anesthesia and Analgesia. 1996;**82**(6):1197-1204

[20] Parnis SJ, Barker DS, Van der Walt JH. Clinical predictors of anaesthetic complications in children with respiratory tract infections. Paediatric Anaesthesia. 2001;**11**(1):29-40

[21] Tait AR, Knight PR. The effects of general anesthesia on upper respiratory tract infections in children. Anesthesiology. 1987;**67**(6):930-935

[22] Coté CJ. The upper respiratory tract infection (URI) dilemma: Fear of a complication or litigation? Anesthesiology. 2001;**95**(2):283-285

[23] Gunawardana RH. Difficult laryngoscopy in cleft lip and palate surgery. British Journal of Anaesthesia. 1996;**76**(6):757-759

[24] Arteau-Gauthier I, Leclerc JE, Godbout A. Can we predict a difficult intubation in cleft lip/palate patients? Journal of Otolaryngology - Head & Neck Surgery. 2011;**40**(5):413-419

[25] Reséndiz-Álvarez Y. Manejo anestésico para pacientes con labio y paladar hendido. Rev Mex Anestesiol. 2015;**38**(Suppl 1):245-246

[26] Kularni KR, Patil MR, Shirke AM, Jadhav SB. Perioperative respiratory complications in cleft lip and palate repair: An audit of 1000 cases under "smile train project". Indian. Indian Journal of Anaesthesia. 2013;**57**:562-568. DOI: 10.4103/0019-5049.123328

[27] Bolton P. Anaesthesia for cleft lip and palate surgery. Anaesthesia and Intensive Care Medicine. 2006;**5**:157. DOI: 10.1383/anes.2006.7.5.157

[28] Jindal P, Khurana G. A retrospective analysis of anesthetic experience in 2917 patients posted for cleft5 lip and palate repair. Anesthesia, Essays and Researches. 2013;**7**(3):350-354. DOI: 10.4103/0259-1162.123233

[29] Takemura H, Yasumoto K, Toi T, Hosoyamada A. Correlation of cleft type with incidence of perioperative respiratory complications in infants with cleft lip and palate. Paediatric Anaesthesia. 2002;**12**(7):585-588

[30] Steinmetz J, Holm-Knudsen R, Sørensen MK, Eriksen K, Rasmussen LS. Hemodynamic differences between propofol-remifentanil and sevoflurane anesthesia for repair of cleft lip and palate in infants. Paediatric Anaesthesia. 2007;**17**(1):32-37. DOI: 10.1111/j.1460-9592.2006.01999.x

[31] Simion C, Corcoran J, Iyer A, Suresh S. Postoperative pain control for primary cleft lip repair in infants: Is there an advantage in performing peripheral nerve blocks? Paediatric Anaesthesia. 2008;**18**(11):1060-1065. DOI: 10.1111/j.1460-9592.2008.02721.x

[32] Feriani G, Hatanaka E, Torloni MR. Da silva EM: Infraorbital nerve block for postoperative pain following cleft lip repair in children. Cochrane Database of Systematic Reviews. 2016;**4**:CD011131. DOI: 10.1002/14651858.CD011131.pub2

[33] Rajamani A, Kamat V, Rajavel VP, Murthy J, Hussain SA. A comparison of bilateral infraorbital nerve block with intravenous fentanyl for analgesia following cleft lip repair in children. Paediatric Anaesthesia. 2007;**17**:133-139. DOI: 10.1111/j.1460-9592.2006.02032.x

[34] Ahuja S, Datta A, Krishna A, Bhattacharya A. Infra-orbital nerve block for relief of postoperative pain following cleft lip surgery in infants. Anaesthesia. 1994;**49**:441-444

[35] Prabhu KP, Wig J, Grewal S. Bilateral infraorbital nerve block is superior to peri-incisional infiltration for analgesia after repair of cleft lip. Scandinavian Journal of Plastic and Reconstructive Surgery and Hand Surgery. 1999;**33**:83-87

[36] Nicodemus HF, Ferrer MJR, Cristobal VC, aI. Bilateral infraorbital block with 0.5% bupivacaine as postoperative analgesia following cheiloplasty in children. Scandinavian Journal of Plastic and Reconstructive Surgery and Hand Surgery. 1991;**25**:253-257

[37] Mesnil M, Dadure C, Captier G, Raux O, Rochette A, Canaud N, Sauter M, Capdevila X. A new approach for peri-operative analgesia of cleft palate repair in infants: The bilateral suprazygomatic maxillary nerve block. Paediatric Anaesthesia. 2010;**20**:343-349. DOI: 10.1111/j.1460-9592.2010.03262.x

[38] Chiono J, Raux O, Bringuier S, et al. Bilateral suprazygomatic maxillary nerve block for cleft palate repair in children: A prospective, randomized, double-blind study versus placebo. Anesthesiology. 2014;**120**(6):1362-1369. DOI: 10.1097/ALN.0000000000000171

[39] Nour C, Ratsiu J, Singh N. Analgesic effectiveness of acetaminophen for primary cleft palate repair in young children: A randomized placebo controlled trial. Paediatric Anaesthesia. 2014;**24**(6):574-581. DOI: 10.1111/pan.12393

[40] Bremerich DH, Neidhart G, Heimann K, Kessler P, Behne M. Prophylactically-administered rectal acetaminophen does not reduce postoperative opioid requirements in infants and small children undergoing elective cleft palate repair. Anesthesia and Analgesia. 2001; **92**(4):907-912

[41] Kayyal TA, Wolfswinkel EM, Weathers WM, et al. Treatment effects of dexmedetomidine and ketamine on postoperative analgesia after cleft palate repair. Craniomaxillofacial Trauma and Reconstruction. 2014;**7**(2):131-138. DOI: 10.1055/s-0034-1371446

[42] Dorfman DW, Ciminello FS, Wong GB. Tongue suture placement after cleft palate repair. The Journal of Craniofacial Surgery. 2010;**21**(5):1601-1603. DOI: 10.1097/SCS.0b013e3181ebccb1

[43] Gallagher S, Ferrera A, Spera L, et al. Utility of tongue stitch and nasal trumpet in the immediate postoperative outcome of cleft palatoplasty. Plastic and Reconstructive Surgery. 2016;**137**(2):569-573. DOI: 10.1097/01.prs.0000475786.60069.a3

[44] Lewis CW, Jacob LS, Lehmann CU. AAP section on oral health: The primary care pediatrician and the care of children with cleft lip and/or cleft palate. Pediatrics. 2017; **139**(5):e20170628. DOI: 10.1542/peds.2017-1921

[45] Maine RG, Hoffman WY, Palacios-Martínez JH, Corlew DS, Gregory GA. Comparison of fistula rates after palatoplasty for international and local surgeons on surgical missions in Ecuador with rates at a craniofacial center in the United States. Plastic and Reconstructive Surgery. 2012;**129**(2):319e-326e. DOI: 10.1097/PRS.0b013e31823aea7e

[46] Schneider WJ, Politis GD, Gosain AK, Migliori MR, Cullington JR, Corlew DS, Wexler AM, Flick R, Van Beek AL. Volunteers in plastic surgery guidelines for providing surgical care for children in the less developed world. Plastic and Reconstructive Surgery. 2011;**127**(6):2477-2486. DOI: 10.1097/PRS.0b013e3182131d2a

Chapter 4

Anesthesia Management for Large-Volume Liposuction

Sergio Granados-Tinajero,
Carlos Buenrostro-Vásquez,
Cecilia Cárdenas-Maytorena and
Marcela Contreras-López

Additional information is available at the end of the chapter

http://dx.doi.org/10.5772/intechopen.83630

Abstract

The apparent easiness with which liposuction is performed favors that patients, young surgeons, and anesthesiologists without experience in this field ignore the many events that occur during this procedure. Liposuction is a procedure to improve the body contour and not a surgery to reduce weight, although recently people who have failed in their plans to lose weight look at liposuction as a means to contour their body figure. Tumescent liposuction of large volumes requires a meticulous selection of each patient; their preoperative evaluation and perioperative management are essential to obtain the expected results. The various techniques of general anesthesia are the most recommended and should be monitored in the usual way, as well as monitoring the total doses of infiltrated local anesthetics to avoid systemic toxicity. The management of intravenous fluids is controversial, but the current trend is the restricted use of hydrosaline solutions. The most feared complications are deep vein thrombosis, pulmonary thromboembolism, fat embolism, lung edema, hypothermia, infections and even death. The adherence to the management guidelines and prophylaxis of venous thrombosis/thromboembolism is mandatory.

Keywords: tumescent liposuction, large volume, anesthesia

1. Introduction

Tumescent liposuction is a cosmetic surgical procedure that consists of a suction-assisted lipoplasty that removes unwanted fat deposited under the skin. Liposuction has its beginnings in 1921, with the Parisian surgeon Charles Dujarrier who was interested in body shaping and fat removal. In 1970s, the technique evolved with various doctors such as Shrudde,

Kesserling and Meyer, the Fischers, and many more. The technique was again modified in 1977 by the French surgeon, Yves Gerard Illouz, who added hyaluronidase and saline solution to try to emulsify the fat and facilitate its aspiration, later called the wet technique [1–3]. It was not until the mid-1980s that the American dermatologist, Klein, described the tumescent technique, in which considerable amounts of sodium chloride solution, local anesthetic, epinephrine, and bicarbonate were infiltrated in the fatty tissue to expand and increase its turgor in order to create a level to facilitate the suction and reduce blood losses [4]. During tumescent liposuction a variable amount of crystalloid solution is infused, including dissolved epinephrine to thicken the subcutaneous fat layer in order to remove the highest possible amount of fat, thus decreasing blood loss to amounts as low as 1% of all the aspirated volume. Lidocaine can be added to the solution to produce local anesthesia during and after the procedure.

Although liposuction appears to be easy and harmless, it is not a trivial procedure because it can potentially involve serious complications like deep vein thrombosis (DVT), pulmonary embolism (PE), pulmonary edema, fat embolism, hypothermia, and even death [3, 5]. A painful recovery is also possible. Large-volume liposuction needs special care to avoid hypothermia, keep an appropriate fluid balance and DVT/PE prophylaxis.

This chapter focuses on large-volume liposuction done under general anesthesia, the most important technical aspects and literature data regarding risks, complications, and anesthesiological considerations.

2. Types of liposuction

According to the infiltration techniques for liposuction, this procedure can be classified into four categories [6]:

1. Dry technique: In which the aspiration cannula is inserted directly into the space from which the fat will be removed without any infiltration of the tissues. The estimated blood losses range from 20 to 45% of the aspirated volume.

2. Wet technique: In relation to the expected amount of aspirated volume, 200–300 ml of solution is injected in each area to be treated. Blood losses are calculated from 4 to 30% of the volume aspirated.

3. Super wet technique: The amount of infiltrated solution (calculated in 1 ml for each ml of the aspirated estimate) is equal to the amount of fat removed. Blood losses are calculated at 1% of the volume aspirated.

4. Tumescent method: A large amount of solution (estimated at 3–4 ml per ml expected to be aspirated) is injected into the fatty tissue, seeking to increase the space occupied by the fat, in addition to giving it a firm and turgid consistency (**Figure 1**). Blood losses are calculated at 1% of the aspirated volume.

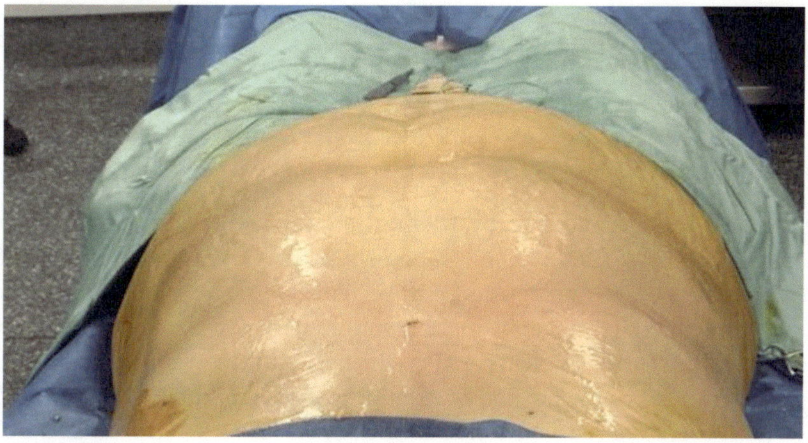

Figure 1. Abdomen infiltrated with 6 liters of tumescent solution. Note the pale coloration of the skin secondary to the effect of injected adrenaline.

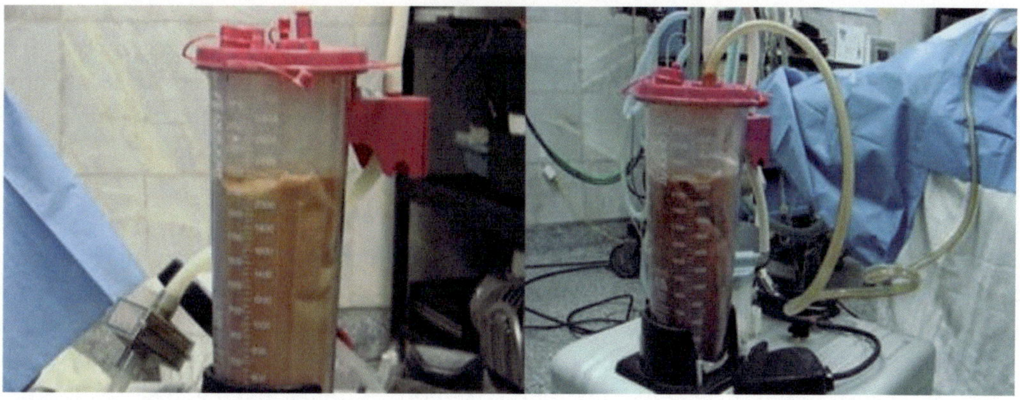

Figure 2. The left image shows little blood compared to the image on the right with a large amount of blood in the liposuction container.

Liposuction can also be classified into two types according to the aspirated volume: large volume (>4 liters aspirated) and low volume (<4 liters aspirated). From here we must always keep in mind that the higher the volume aspirated, almost inevitably a greater amount of tumescent solution will have to be infiltrated in the dermoclysis. As this volume of infiltration increases, so does the risk of causing pulmonary edema, for which in these conditions the management of intravenous fluids must be very cautious, always tending to the restriction both in the transoperative period and in the first hours of postanesthetic recovery (**Figure 2**).

According to the surgical instruments used, liposuction is called power-assisted, laser-assisted, or ultrasonic-assisted lipoplasty. Manual liposuction using different sizes of syringes is a technique that is still used for small areas.

3. Tumescent solutions

Currently, the most used solution to generate the tumescence is the one described by Klein [4, 7], and a more reasonable variant—which we prefer to use but little is known—is the one proposed by Hunstad [8, 9], as seen in **Table 1**.

In the tumescent solution described by Klein, the local anesthetic was diluted in isotonic saline solution. However, when isotonic saline solution is used as a diluent, if the patient is not under anesthesia, a burn sensation will be reported as the solution is infiltrated. It is reasonably recommended that when using this solution, the acidic pH of the 0.9% saline solution should be neutralized with bicarbonate, which in addition reduces pain; by increasing the pH, it also increases the proportion of non-ionized lipid soluble lidocaine, which favors a faster entry into the nerve cell where lidocaine acts. When lactate Ringer's solution is used, this burning sensation does not occur upon infiltration, and the sodium load is reduced. It should be noted that the dose of lidocaine and epinephrine should be regulated according to the maximum doses to be considered as safe.

Regarding the local anesthetics used, there are reports with articaine or prilocaine. Liposuction done with up to 38.2 mg/kg bodyweight of articaine HCl produced plasmatic concentrations as high as 1719–7292 ng/mL, without symptoms of systemic toxicity which could be explained by the rapid hydrolysis through the plasmatic esterases. These data show that articaine is safe for infiltration during liposuction [10]. The groups that have reported the use of prilocaine have not detected elevated levels of it in plasma or methemoglobinemia [11, 12], although Yildirim et al. described a patient with 40% methemoglobinemia that developed 8 h after liposuction was performed with almost 1000 mg of prilocaine [13]. In our surgical facility, the most used local anesthetic is lidocaine, and even though for other applications when used in association with epinephrine, the maximum limit is established at 7 mg/kg. In the specific case of the tumescent solution for liposuction, the safety range is 35–55 mg/kg [14, 15]. We prefer to stay at the lower limit of 35 mg/kg in order to be more cautious, given that since the surgical team does not keep accurate control of the injected lidocaine or takes into consideration possible drug interactions or special conditions of the patient. The concentrations of lidocaine vary according to the vascularity of the area in which the liposuction is to be performed. In more sensitive or vascularized areas such as the chest and abdomen, the concentration or amount of local anesthetic mass can be increased and decreased in less sensitive areas such as the thighs.

Klein solution	**Hunstad solution**
1000 mL isotonic saline solution	1000 mL Ringer's lactate solution
50 mL, 1% lidocaine	50 mL lidocaine 1%
1 mL (1: 1000 epinephrine)	1 mL (1: 1000 epinephrine)
12.5 mL (8.4% sodium bicarbonate)	

Table 1. Tumescent solution.

Lidocaine toxicity is in function if the peak plasma concentration is reached, which will depend on several factors such as the total amount of mg/kg, as well as its rate of absorption and elimination, so that the peak levels of lidocaine and its active metabolite (monoethylglycinexylidide) occur in a period as variable as 8–32 h after infiltration has been done. For this reason alone, for patients who are treated with this procedure, it is not recommended to do it in an outpatient setting, because the maximum concentrations of lidocaine and its active metabolite will most often take the patient at home with little vigilance.

Lidocaine is eliminated from the body by diethylation in the liver by isoenzyme groups 1A2 and 3A4 of cytochrome p450. Thus, all drugs that inhibit isoenzyme 3A4 and cytochrome P450 can affect the metabolism of lidocaine. For this reason, lidocaine doses should be reduced in patients who use medications that interfere with the cytochrome P450 system or that affect the hepatic blood flow. The factors that can modify the systemic absorption of lidocaine need to be considered. Obviously, the reached concentration of the drug, the degree of vascularity of the infiltrated tissue, the concomitant use of vasoconstrictor drugs, and the infiltration rate [3] are very important.

The adequate use of epinephrine in the tumescent solution theoretically allows blood loss to be 1–2% of the total volume aspirated. The maximum recommended total dose of epinephrine is 0.07 mg/kg. Vasoconstrictors are used to reduce blood circulation in the tissues, which helps to slow the absorption of local anesthetics. Adrenaline is the most commonly used vasoconstrictor; the recommended concentration for the tumescent solution ranges from 0.25 to 1 mg/Lt, depending on the tissue vascularity in question. In more vascularized tissues, the recommended concentration is 1 mg/L to be decreased to 0.5 mg/L in body areas with less vascularization (**Figure 3**). If it is anticipated that this maximum dose will be exceeded, the procedure

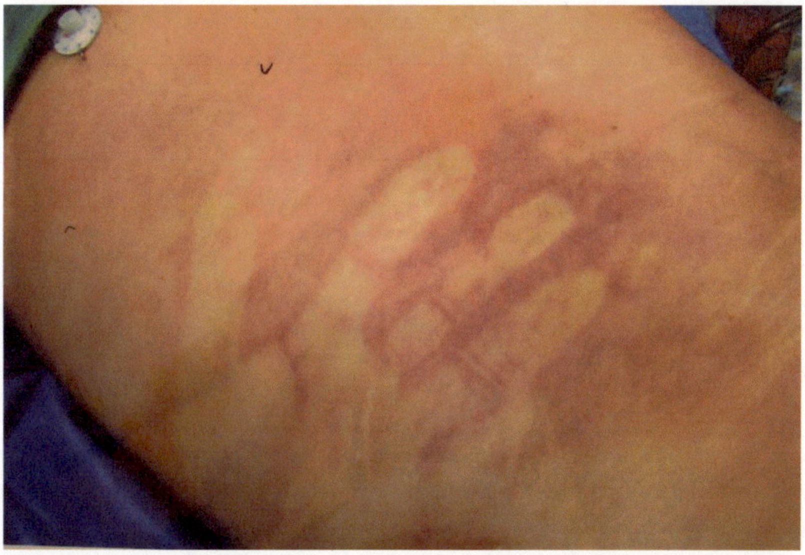

Figure 3. Infiltrated back. Note the changes in skin circulation due to the tumescent solution, with a marked delay in capillary refill.

should be done replacing the adrenaline with other options such as 1-ornithine-8-vasopressin in concentrations of 0.01 IU/ml, with the disadvantage of having to use it in unheated solution with the consequent hypothermia of the patient.

4. Preoperative evaluation

Although it is well established that liposuction is not a treatment for obesity, more often than desired, the obese patient is programed for this type of procedure, and there are usually other associated comorbidities such as high blood pressure, diabetes mellitus, metabolic syndrome, ischemic heart disease, DVT, and obstructive sleep apnea. If despite recognizing that liposuction is not a reasonable treatment for obesity, if in any case it is decided to do this procedure, the minimum required is that, in the case of hypertension and diabetes, these conditions should be well controlled (it is advisable to postpone patients who have recently changed medications or doses in order to avoid unpleasant outcomes). If the risk of DVT, consider pharmacological thromboprophylaxis apart from mechanical prophylactic measures.

It is common that this type of patients is using recognized or unrecognized (natural remedies) medications and "herbal aids" to lose weight. This type of drugs ranges from amphetamines, thyroid hormones and ephedrine and a fairly large list of herbs and teas that if we take the care to inquire about it (identify them and look for their pharmacological effects), we will find that at least they alter the coagulation system or facilitate the interactions with epinephrine (see Chapter 1). Therefore, the patient should be instructed to suspend all this type of medications and naturopathic remedies at least 2 weeks before surgery. Needless to say, it is a contraindicated procedure in cocaine addicts.

With regard to laboratory tests, in our work center, it seems that it is exaggerated, but the type of patients and the procedures that are carried out have led us to request complete blood chemistry, basic metabolic panel, quantification of glycosylated hemoglobin (if the patient is diabetic), thyroid profile, coagulation times, liver function tests, pregnancy detection, serological detection of hepatitis A, B, and C, as well as detection of antibodies against HIV. If the patient presents some suspicious data, antidoping is added. All patients, regardless of their age, undergo ECG [6].

5. Preanesthetic medication

The preanesthetic medication in this group of patients is an important part of the preoperative management and should include not only sedative and hypnotic drugs but also an effective scheme that prevents the possibility of emesis and postoperative pain with neuropathic characteristics, which is secondary to multiple nervous fiber trauma of medium and small caliber. A typical preanesthetic scheme is lorazepam, dexamethasone, ondansetron, gabapentin, or pregabalin. A nonsteroidal anti-inflammatory analgesic can be added.

6. Anesthesia management

While liposuction of large volumes can be done with any anesthesia technique, we strongly recommend the use of general anesthesia. The anesthetic induction is done in the usual way, being propofol the most used drug. For muscular relaxation for endotracheal intubation, a non-depolarizing drug with rapid action such as rocuronium or atracurium, although vecuronium is probably the most used muscle relaxants due to its safety and low cost. For the maintenance of anesthesia, desflurane, sevoflurane or isoflurane alone or in combination with opioids can be used. Ketofol have been recommended by several authors. Muscle relaxation is optional during the surgery.

In our experience, which is worth taking into consideration, since in the last 8 years, we have accumulated an average of 200 large-volume liposuctions per year (with the peculiarity that it is the same surgeon and the same anesthesiologist). We usually premedicate patients with ranitidine, metoclopramide, ondansetron, and the prophylactic antibiotic of the surgeon's choice. Induction is with fentanyl 3–4 mμ/kg and vecuronium to facilitate orotracheal intubation (usually 4–6 mg) and propofol 2 mg/kg. We continue with inhalatory anesthesia with low flows, in general terms only use oxygen 350 to maximum 400 mL/minute, and desflurane given its faster response to modify the desired CAM. As approximately 60–70% of the time, the procedure will be done with the patient facing down, more when it includes lipoinjection in the buttocks. The patient is intubated orotracheally with a spiral reinforced cuffed tracheal tube (like Sheridan Spiral-Flex®) properly fixed. We never relied on a laryngeal mask; no matter the discussion, it will never approach the security provided by an endotracheal tube. Due to the situation of changes in the patient's position, experience is necessary in turning the patient from supine to the ventral position and ventral to the supine, protecting the cervical spine and ensuring that the endotracheal tube does not move. It is necessary to have protection devices for pressure points, which allows us to keep the patient upside down, taking care of pressure points on the nose and eyes fundamentally (**Figure 4**) [16].

The patient scheduled for liposuction at least qualifies as a moderate thromboembolic risk, so all of them must have compression stockings and intermittent pneumatic compression systems installed, both during surgery and during all the time that they remain in the clinic or at least until they start ambulation. In special cases of higher risk, pharmacological thromboprophylaxis with low-molecular-weight heparin is necessary.

As for the monitoring equipment, beyond the required pulse oximetry, ECG with automated analysis of the ST segment, noninvasive blood pressure measurement every 5 minutes, capnography, and analysis of inhaled and exhaled gases, if available. As for temperature monitoring is useful to keep the record in two channels, central and peripheral temperature, since the isolated reading of the peripheral is of little use, it is more advisable to have both readings and be aware of the gap between the two. Although we have neuromuscular relaxation monitor, given the type of surgery, the low doses of the neuromuscular blocking agents injected for the tracheal intubation and its pharmacokinetic profile, at the end of the surgery, have no residual effects. BIS or entropy monitor can be very useful, given that the hemodynamic variations of the patients are not rare as a result of the adrenergic stimuli due to the infiltrated

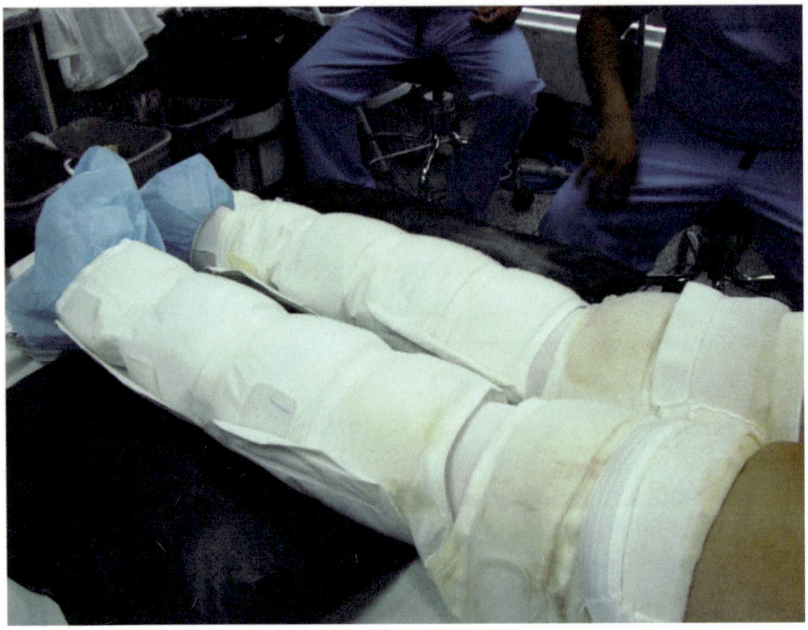

Figure 4. Proper mechanical thromboprophylaxis by compression stockings and intermittent pneumatic compression system in lower limbs.

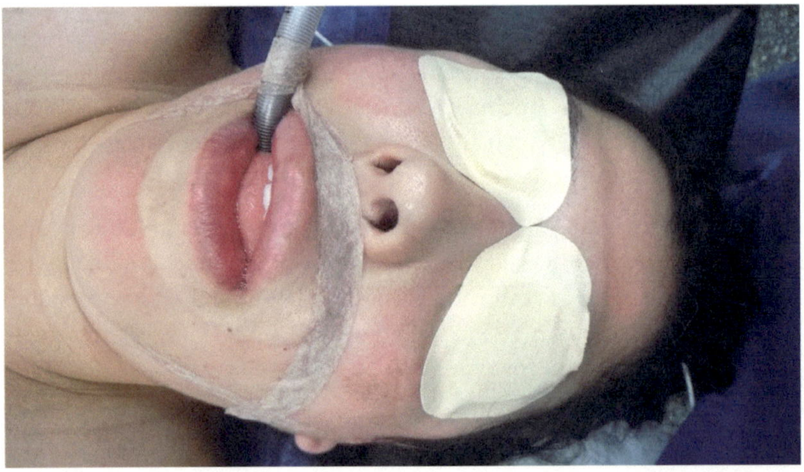

Figure 5. Hyperemia is seen in the areas of the face where the device for protecting the nose and eyes rested, as well as adequate eye occlusion.

epinephrine and that they do not necessarily have to do with the need of changing the anesthetic depth (**Figure 5**).

One of the reasons to use general anesthesia is because through endotracheal intubation and mechanical ventilation, it is easy to control the respiratory function more efficiently. In this sense, spirometry has great importance. If you do not use spirometry with these types of procedures, you could say that you ventilate blindly, considering the almost obliged obesity of many of

http://dx.doi.org/10.5772/intechopen.83630

these patients, in which their thoracic dynamics differ with just the change to ventral position. Normally, we ventilate the patients with volume-controlled mode, calculating their tidal volume between 6 and 7 mL/kg, and always keep a sequential record of the peak pressure reached with these volumes. In many patients, with only the change to ventral position, the peak pressure increases between 2 and 4 cm H_2O, values that increase even more when the tumescence is completed either from the back or the abdomen. The vast majority of patients tolerate it adequately, but between 5 and 10% present a peak pressure increase that forces us to consider that all the extra effort that the ventilator is generating is what helps meet those required volumes. A patient with upper spinal block, in ventral position, sedated and with a nasal cannula, definitely cannot meet the required ventilatory work. Sometimes it is better to change to a pressure-controlled mode, usually lowering to maximum pressures of 18–20 cm H_2O, but always observing the expiratory volume, so that it is sufficient to maintain an adequate reading of CO_2ET, maintaining adequate alveolar ventilation without the significant increase in airway pressure that can be generated in volume-controlled mode (**Figures 6** and **7**).

As mentioned before, it is mandatory to supervise the cumulative dose of lidocaine to avoid systemic toxicity; it must be taken in mind that although it is being used within the limits recommended as safe, it must be considered that its enzymatic metabolism depends on cytochrome P450, which is also responsible for the metabolism of other drugs. This could cause the 3A4 subfamily of cytochrome P450 to be saturated and alter the metabolism of lidocaine. Midazolam competes in its metabolism in this subgroup, which could decrease the elimination of lidocaine, and with its effects, midazolam may mask the toxicity symptoms of lidocaine up until the onset of cardiovascular collapse. Other drugs that inhibit the 3A4 subfamily of cytochrome P450 are listed in **Table 2** [17, 18]. As it is observed, the list is quite extensive, making it difficult to have in mind all these possible interactions, the reason why we recommend the online use of the system of detection of interactions and undesirable side effects "epocartes."

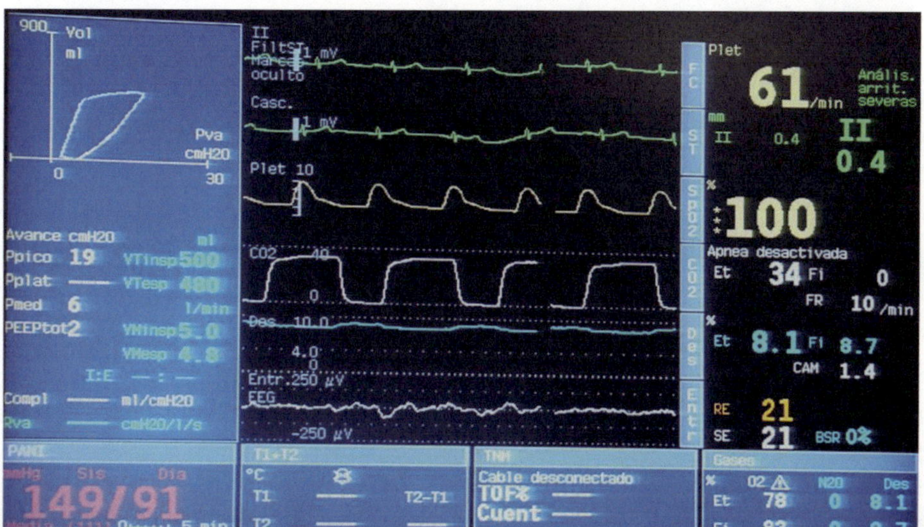

Figure 6. Observe the adequate anesthetic depth (entropy readings) despite the rise in blood pressure secondary to epinephrine infiltration.

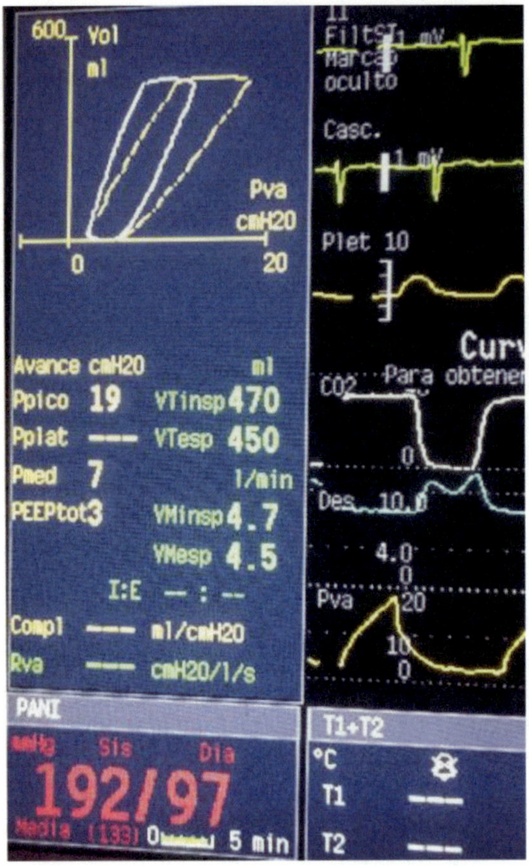

Figure 7. Increase of blood pressure during the infiltration of the solution for tumescence in a hypertensive patient. In the upper part of the figure in yellow, we can see the current loop of spirometry, produced by the decrease in thoracic compliance, compared with the reference white loop before infiltration.

Propofol	**Methylprednisolone**	**Amiodarone**
Flunitrazepam	Dexamethasone	Verapamil
Diazepam	Itraconozole	Atenolol
Triazolam	Ketoconazole	Labetalol
Paroxetine	Miconazole	Pindolol
Carbamazepine	Fluconazole	Propranolol
Fluoxetine	Isoniazid	Metoprolol
Sertraline	Clarithromycin	Diltiazem
Nefazodone	Chloramphenicol	Nicardipine
Terfenadine	Erythromycin	Timolol
Methadone	Tetracycline	Nadolol
Danazol	Cimetidine	Nifedipine
Thyroxine	Quinidine	Pentoxifylline

Table 2. Drugs that inhibit the 3A4 subfamily of cytochrome P450.

7. Management of perioperative intravenous fluids

For safety reasons, tumescent liposuction of large volumes is a surgery in which patients must stay at least 1 night hospitalized in an environment that guarantees their monitoring and safety. Often, there are patients who want extensive liposuction that can be as much as 30% of their total body surface, the remaining 70% will stay on the infiltrated tissues, and from there it will be reabsorbed, with the potential for fluid overload. Although the perioperative management of liquids during liposuction remains an unresolved controversy, especially in liposuction of large volumes, the current trend is to decrease the administration of liquids and sodium to avoid fluid overload, pulmonary edema, and congestive heart failure.

A recent study was done in China by Wang et al. [19], who retrospectively reviewed 83 medical records of patients who underwent extensive liposuction under intravenous monitored sedation with propofol 1–2 mg/kg/h and remifentanil 1–7 μg/kg/h. The intraoperative fluid ratio was 1.66 for extensive liposuction. These authors did not find cases of pulmonary edema, congestive heart failure, or other important complications. The average diuresis in the operating room, the recovery room, and in the surgical floors was 1.35, 2.3, and 1.4 mL/kg/h, respectively. The administration of intravenous fluids during liposuction decreased approximately 300–500 mL. The total volume of intravenous injection was also reduced to less than 1500 mL when the patient was in the recovery room and on the floor of the hospital. The Colombian Consensus recommends to consider the effect of dermoclysis of the tumescent solutions that are injected to the patients [20].

The liposuction removes approximately 30% of the infused tumescent solution, so for each liter of infiltrated tumescent solution, 700 mL are absorbed, so they should be considered as part of the fluids administered to the patient.

Another piece of information that can be used as a guide is to administer intravenous crystalloid solutions from 0.1 to 0.25 mL per mL of aspirate [21, 22].

8. Risks and complications

Liposuction risks and complications are undervalued and underreported. When analyzing the medical literature related to the subject, it is always necessary to take into consideration the context from which the experiences are taken, since it is very different to perform liposuction of low volumes than liposuction of high volumes. In this way, there are interesting publications [23] but refer to cosmetic surgery performed in the office, for which the following possible contraindications are mentioned:

- Liposuction >5 liters
- Tumescent solution >5 liters
- Liposuction of large volumes with a second procedure
- Multiple procedures including abdominoplasty
- Anticipated blood loss >500 mL in adults
- Duration of surgery >6 h

Risks associated with tumescent infiltration and liposuction include DVT/PE, fatty embolism, anemia, perforation of the abdominal wall, pleural perforation, infection, fluid overload, pulmonary edema, hypothermia, and toxicity by local anesthetics and epinephrine. It is quite important to consider the necessary care during changes in position (ventral decubitus to prone decubitus) to minimize hemodynamic changes when patients are turned around and protect certain areas to avoid pressure injuries, corneal injuries, neural damage, and even blindness after anesthesia surgery. A recent report [24] mentioned the five more frequent serious complications of liposuction: thromboembolic disease, fat embolism, pulmonary edema, lidocaine intoxication, and intraabdominal visceral lesion. These events are easily preventable by simple measurements and safety protocols. The literature is full of reports of complicated patients during or after liposuction, and it is enough to mention some of these complications to encourage specialized care and stay within the recommended guidelines.

8.1. Deep vein thrombosis and embolism

Abdominoplasty is the plastic surgery procedure with the highest incidence of death secondary to PE. In addition, it must be considered that if the abdominoplasty is associated with liposuction of large volumes, the risk of PE increases. It is estimated that the rate of thromboembolism if these procedures are combined increases 6.6 times. The rate of nonlethal PE was 8.8% in patients who had an abdominoplasty with wide resection, combined with liposuction with surgical times of more than 140 minutes [25]. The causes that increase the risk of PE are the mechanical factors that favor blood stagnation in the lower extremities, such as the surgical position, abdominal compression, and the use of bandages and garments in the postoperative period [26]. In a survey conducted by the American Society of Plastic and Esthetic Surgery, a mortality of 1 for 47,415 liposuctions was reported, 1 for 7314 if liposuction was combined with other procedures, and 1 for 3281 when liposuction had been combined with abdominoplasty; this is 14 times greater than with liposuction alone [27]. Ibarra et al. [20] contributed to the elaboration of the Consensus of the Colombian Society of Anesthesiology and Resuscitation (SCARE) and of the Colombian Society of Plastic Surgery on the recommendations for the management of low-risk elective patients. Within this consensus, the following measures are mentioned: prevention of DVT, comfortable position (legs in partial flexion of knees and extremities), intermittent pneumatic compression during surgery and until discharge. Elastic compression stockings from the preoperative period until ambulation are mandatory (**Figure 8**).

Consider the use of low-molecular-weight heparin every 12 h until ambulation is normal. The following should be considered for patients with increased risk of DVT: patients with a history of previous episode of DVT, patients undergoing procedures lasting more than 5 h, patients with liposuction of large volumes (>5 liters), patients who undergo combined procedures that include abdominoplasty, patients who arrive in cities of high altitude (>2000 m asl) 2 or less days before surgery, patients traveling in the immediate preoperative or aspire to travel with a duration of 4 h or more within the first week of the postoperative period, and the patients who undergo gluteal lipoinjections.

Morales and his group studied the prophylactic effect of rivaroxaban and apixaban in patients undergoing liposuction of large volumes and other body contouring procedures, finding

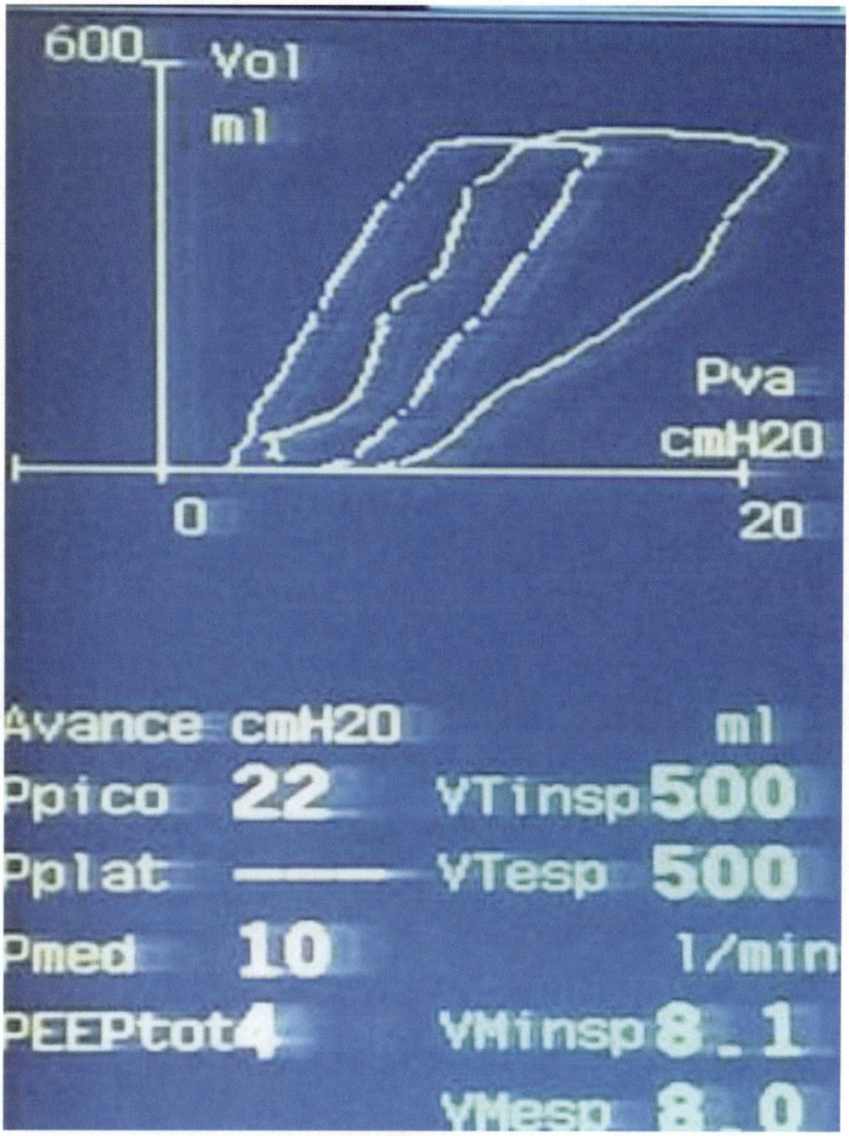

Figure 8. Comparison of spirometry loops, the basal with a peak pressure of the airway of 15 cm of water, and the second obtained once the patient's back has been infiltrated, rising to 22 cm of water.

that their thromboprophylactic effects and side effects are similar to each other and to low-molecular-weight heparin [28].

8.2. Anemia

Anemia is a frequent postoperative complication in patients undergoing liposuction, especially in liposuction of large volumes. The use of vasopressors in the tumescent solutions that are injected into the fatty tissue at the beginning of this procedure decreases bleeding due to vasoconstriction, although there are some areas such as the torso and neck where bleeding is usually more abundant. Cansancao et al. [29] administered 10 mg/kg of intravenous tranexamic acid preoperative and postoperative vs. placebo in patients undergoing liposuction. The volume of blood loss for every liter of lipoaspirate was 56.2% less in the tranexamic group compared with the control group ($p < 0.001$). Hematocrit levels at day 7 postoperatively were 48% less in group 1 compared with group 2 ($p = 0.001$). Furthermore, a 1% drop in the hematocrit level was found after liposuction of 812 ± 432 ml in group 1 and 379 ± 204 ml in group 2. The authors concluded that tranexamic acid could allow for aspiration of 114% more fat, with comparable variation in hematocrit levels. Although erythropoietin has been used to improve anemia after liposuction and decrease the frequency of hemotransfusions, its usefulness has not been demonstrated [30]. It is advisable to check the hematocrit value before discharging the patient; in our patients, the hemoglobin values obtained by co-oximetry have a good correlation with the values obtained by the laboratory.

8.3. Drug interactions

Take care of possible drug interactions including natural products and anabolic steroids. Clarify in informed consent the high risk of interaction of substances such as cocaine, amphetamines, ecstasy, and other recreational drugs, with anesthetic and vasoactive medications. In suspected cases, antidoping and toxicology tests can be done [20].

Liposuction of large volumes is associated with important hemodynamic alterations: an increase in the cardiac index, heart rate, mean arterial pressure of the pulmonary, ejection volume index, and right ventricular work index are observed as well as a decrease in mean arterial pressure. Epinephrine, which is usually used at considerable doses during liposuction, may be responsible for tachycardia and increased cardiac index. The decrease in mean arterial pressure and systemic vascular resistance is probably due to the effects of general anesthesia and opioids in the transoperative period, but also the reduction of peripheral vascular resistance may be due to the dominant action of the epinephrine on the beta2 receptors of skeletal muscle vessels, where an increase in blood flow is observed.

8.4. Hypothermia

There is an increased risk of hypothermia in patients of large volume liposuction since there are large areas of body surface exposed to temperature loss. If the anesthesiologist does not insist, the nursing staff tends not to adequately heat the dermoclysis solutions, or if the surgeon has no experience or does not care about hypothermia, he/she can make the procedure excessively long, without considering that regardless of the type of anesthesia, this will always help to facilitate hypothermia. It is necessary to maintain the temperature of the operating room, even in hot climates in no less than 25°C or 77°F, even if it goes against the surgeon's comfort and other operating room staff. We must bear in mind the complications that hypothermia can cause, such as cardiac dysrhythmias, coagulopathies, oliguria, and electrolyte imbalance and an important increase in the consumption of oxygen during the chill phase. Both the hemodynamic changes and the tendency to hypothermia persist at least in the first 24 h of the postoperative [31].

8.5. Fat embolism

Fat embolism and fat embolism syndrome are another serious complication whose incidence is not known, but apparently has increased [32]. Fat embolisms are fat drops that enter the circulatory system, typically after trauma, that may or may not lead to the development of fat embolism syndrome, a rare and ill-defined diagnosis that can cause multiorgan failure and death. Fat embolism syndrome is defined as the entry of fat into the blood circulation with a clinical pattern characterized by hypoxemia, respiratory failure, neurological deterioration, and petechiae that occur in the appropriate clinical context; it is a continuum of fat embolism [33–35]. A study in 30 Wistar rats showed that there was an increased risk of systemic fat embolism in the animals that underwent liposuction-lipoinjection compared to those who only underwent liposuction (3/10 vs. 6/10, respectively). Fat embolism was not detected in rats that were only anesthetized [36]. There is no specific treatment for fat embolism syndrome, therefore prevention is so important as well as prompt detection, and supportive therapy are critical. Most patients with fat embolism or fat embolism syndrome are undiagnosed or misdiagnosed, so their mortality is very high. Most of these cases are diagnosed at autopsy [34].

8.6. Miscellaneous complications

The literature is full of varied reports of complicated patients during or after liposuction, and it is enough to mention some of these complications to encourage specialized care and stay within the recommended guidelines. There is a wide spectrum on liposuction complications: pleural and lung injury, bilothorax, bowel herniation, hematoma, seroma, lymphedema, and abdominal wall injury with damage to intra-abdominal viscera such as the liver, biliary tract, intestinal, or bladder perforation necrotizing fasciitis, blindness, and coronary fat embolism [37–39].

The main risk factors for the development of complications are deficient standards of hygiene, infiltration of multiple liters of wetting solution, prompt postoperative discharge, and selection of unfit patients, lack of surgical anesthesia experience, and early identification of developing complications [40].

9. Postoperative analgesia and hyperbaric oxygen therapy

Postoperative analgesics are extraordinarily mandatory in the professional management and prevention of acute and chronic pain after liposuction. It is usually started from the beginning of the surgery with an infusion with 300 mg of ketorolac, 300 mg of tramadol in 100 mL/2 mL/h, considered as basal analgesic scheme. It is also valid to resort if necessary to some rescue strategies, in which the analgesic and anti-inflammatory effect of hyperbaric oxygenation therapy can be considered. This therapy is routinely provided to all of our patients in the next 4 to 5 days after their procedure [41, 42].

The use of hyperbaric oxygenation therapy (**Figure 9**) has also reduced the need for pharmacological thromboprophylaxis, since it has been shown that hyperbaric oxygen by the action of nitric oxide decreases the expression of intracellular adhesion molecules (ICAM-1),

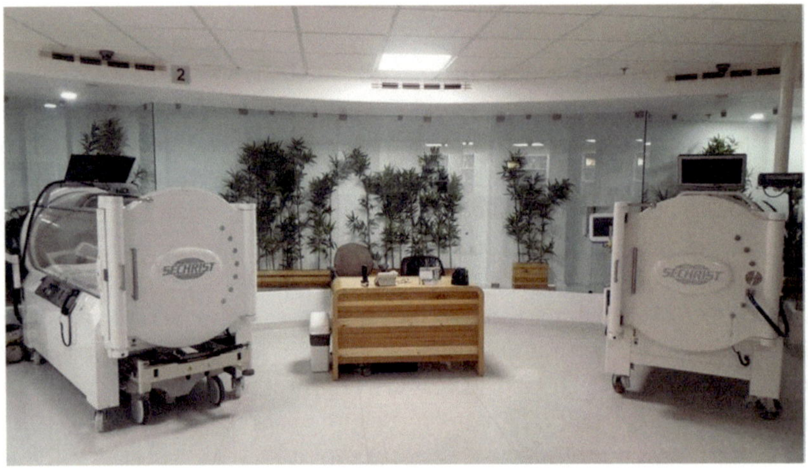

Figure 9. Partial view of the Hyperbaric Center at Buenrostro Clinic of Plastic Surgery and Hyperbaric Medicine in Tijuana México.

a factor that participates in favoring thrombus formation [43]. In addition, another of the already proven actions of hyperbaric oxygen that contribute to diminish the possibility of venous thrombosis formation is its capacity to favor the expression of fibrinolytic factors [44]. In this way in the last 8 years, with an average of 200 liposuctions performed per year, we have only resorted to the use of low-molecular-weight heparin in 2 patients, one of them had a history of deep vein thrombosis 3 years before liposuction, and the other patient was an exceptional case, since for traumatic reasons the patient was paraplegic for 5 years before her surgery.

10. Conclusion

Currently there are many controversies in the selection and better management of patients undergoing liposuction, especially in tumescent liposuction of large volumes. Meticulous selection of each patient is the basis of success, as well as a strategy of prophylaxis of catastrophic events such as thromboembolism, fat embolism, anemia, fluid overload, and infections, among others. Anesthesia is a determining factor and although various anesthesia techniques can be used, we propose general anesthesia as a safe procedure. Hyperbaric oxygenation is an unexploited resource that requires further study in this field.

Acknowledgements

We thank Dr. Victor Whizar-Lugo for his support in updating this chapter.

Conflict of interest

None.

Author details

Sergio Granados-Tinajero[1]*, Carlos Buenrostro-Vásquez[1], Cecilia Cárdenas-Maytorena[2] and Marcela Contreras-López[3]

*Address all correspondence to: granadosts@gmail.com

1 Clínica Buenrostro de Cirugía Plástica y Medicina Hiperbárica, Tijuana, Baja California, México

2 Lotus Med Group, Tijuana, Baja California, México

3 Anesthesia Department, Hospital General de Tijuana, ISESALUD, Tijuana, Baja California, México

References

[1] Schlarb D. Liposuction. Der Hautarzt. 2018;**69**(2):165-176. DOI: 10.1007/s00105-017-4108-z

[2] Bellini E, Grieco MP, Raposio E. A journey through liposuction and liposculture: Review. Annals of Medicine and Surgery (London). 2017;**24**:53-60. DOI: 10.1016/j.amsu.2017.10.024

[3] Sterodimas A, Boriani F, Magarakis E, Nicaretta B, Pereira LH, Illouz YG. Thirty four years of liposuction: Past, present and future. European Review for Medical and Pharmacological Sciences. 2012;**16**(3):393-406

[4] Klein JA. The tumescent technique for liposuction surgery. American Journal of Cosmetic Surgery. 1987;**4**:1124-1132

[5] Tumescent liposuction. Minnesota Department of Health. http://www.health.state.mn.us/htac/lipo.htm Mayo del 2002

[6] Sood J, Jayaraman L, Sethi N. Liposuction: Anaesthesia challenges. Indian Journal of Anaesthesia. 2011;**55**:220-227

[7] Klein JA. Tumescent technique for local anesthesia improves safety in large-volume liposuction. Plastic and Reconstructive Surgery. 1993;**92**:1085-1098

[8] Hunstad JP. Tumescent and syringe liposculpture: A logical partnership. Aesthetic Plastic Surgery. 1995;**19**(4):321-333

[9] Hunstad JP, Aitken ME. Liposuction and tumescent surgery. Clinics in Plastic Surgery. 2006;**33**(1):39-46

[10] Grossmann M, Sattler G, Pistner H, Oertel R, Richter K, Schinzel S, et al. Pharmacokinetics of articaine hydrochloride in tumescent local anesthesia for liposuction. Journal of Clinical Pharmacology. 2004;**44**(11):1282-1289

[11] Augustin M, Maier K, Sommer B, Sattler G, Herberger K. Double-blind, randomized, intraindividual comparison study of the efficacy of prilocaine and lidocaine in tumescent local anesthesia. Dermatology. 2010;**221**(3):248-252. DOI: 10.1159/000319753

[12] Lindenblatt N, Belusa L, Tiefenbach B, Schareck W, Olbrisch RR. Prilocaine plasma levels and methemoglobinemia in patients undergoing tumescent liposuction involving less than 2000 ml. Aesthetic Plastic Surgery. 2004;**28**(6):435-440

[13] Yildirim B, Karagoz U, Acar E, Beydilli H, Nese Yeniceri E, Tanriverdi O, et al. A case report of prilocaine-induced methemoglobinemia after liposuction procedure. Case Reports in Emergency Medicine. 2015;**2015**:282347. DOI: 10.1155/2015/282347

[14] Ostad A, Kageyama N, Moy RL. Tumescent anesthesia with a lidocaine dose of 55 mg/kg is safe for liposuction. Dermatologic Surgery. 1996;**22**(11):921-927

[15] Klein JA, Jeske DR. Estimated maximal safe dosages of tumescent lidocaine. Anesthesia and Analgesia. 2016;**122**(5):1350-1359. DOI: 10.1213/ANE.0000000000001119

[16] Buenrostro-Vásquez C, Buck-Soltero JA, Morales-Valle LA, Granados-Tinajero SO. Anestesia en liposucción de grandes volúmenes. Anest Méx. 2017;(Suppl 1):64-76

[17] Wang G, Cao WG, Zhao TL. Fluid management in extensive liposuction: A retrospective review of 83 consecutive patients. Medicine (Baltimore). 2018;**97**(41):e12655. DOI: 10.1097/MD.0000000000012655

[18] Becker DE. Adverse drug interactions. Anesthesia Progress. 2011;**58**(1):31-41. DOI: 10.2344/0003-3006-58.1.31

[19] Becker DE, Reed KL. Local anesthetics: Review of pharmacological considerations. Anesthesia Progress. 2012;**59**(2):90-101; quiz 102-3. DOI: 10.2344/0003-3006-59.2.90

[20] Ibarra P, Arango J, Bayter J, Castro J, Cortés J, Lascano M, et al. Consenso de la Sociedad Colombiana de Anestesiología y Reanimación, SCARE, y de la Sociedad Colombiana de Cirugía Plástica sobre las recomendaciones para el manejo de pacientes electivos de bajo riesgo. Revista Colombiana de Anestesiología. 2010;**37**:390-403

[21] Trott et al. Safety considerations and fluid resuscitation in liposuction: an analysis of 53 consecutive patients. Plastic and Reconstructive Surgery. 1998;**102**(6):2220-2229

[22] Gilliland MD, Coates N. Tumescent liposuction complicated by pulmonary edema. Plastic and Reconstructive Surgery. 1997;**99**(1):215-219

[23] Bogan V. Anesthesia and safety considerations for office-based cosmetic surgery practice. AANA Journal. 2012;**80**:299-305

[24] Cárdenas-Camarena L, Andrés Gerardo LP, Durán H, Bayter-Marin JE. Strategies for reducing fatal complications in liposuction. Plastic and Reconstructive Surgery. Global Open. 2017;**5**(10):e1539. DOI: 10.1097/GOX.0000000000001539

[25] Gravante G, Araco A, Sorge R, et al. Pulmonary embolism after combined abdominoplasty and flank liposuction: A correlation with the amount of fat removed. Annals of Plastic Surgery. 2008;**60**(6):604-608

[26] Venturi ML, Davison SP, Caprini JA. Prevention of venous thromboembolism in the plastic surgery patient: Current guidelines and recommendations. Aesthetic Surgery Journal. 2009;**29**(5):421-428

[27] Hughes CE III. Reduction of lipoplasty risks and mortality: An ASAPS survey. Aesthetic Surgery Journal. 2001;**21**:120-127

[28] Morales R Jr, Ruff E, Patronella C, Mentz H 3rd, Newall G, Hustak KL, et al. Safety and efficacy of novel oral anticoagulants vs low molecular weight heparin for thromboprophylaxis in large-volume liposuction and body contouring procedures. Aesthetic Surgery Journal. 2016;**36**(4):440-449. DOI: 10.1093/asj/sjv243

[29] Cansancao AL, Condé-Green A, David JA, Cansancao B, Vidigal RA. Use of tranexamic acid to reduce blood loss in liposuction. Plastic and Reconstructive Surgery. 2018;**141**(5):1132-1135. DOI: 10.1097/PRS.0000000000004282

[30] Rosique RG, Rosique MJ, Rabelo MQ. Does postoperative erythropoietin reduce transfusions and hemodynamic instability following liposuction, either alone or associated with abdominoplasty or mammaplasty? A comparative, prospective study of 50 consecutive patients. Aesthetic Plastic Surgery. 2017;**41**(1):98-101. DOI: 10.1007/s00266-016-0748-0

[31] Kenkel JM, Lipschitz AH, Luby M, Kallmeyer I, Sorokin E, Appelt E, et al. Hemodynamic physiology and thermoregulation in liposuction. Plastic and Reconstructive Surgery. 2004;**114**:503-513

[32] Durán H, Cárdenas-Camarena L, Bayter-Marin JE, Ramos-Gallardo G, Robles-Cervantes JA. Microscopic and macroscopic fat embolism: Solving the puzzle with case reports. Plastic and Reconstructive Surgery. 2018;**142**(4):569e-577e. DOI: 10.1097/PRS.0000000000004810

[33] Fukumoto LE, Fukumoto KD. Fat embolism syndrome. The Nursing Clinics of North America. 2018;**53**(3):335-347. DOI: 10.1016/j.cnur.2018.04.003

[34] Cantu CA, Pavlisko EN. Liposuction-induced fat embolism syndrome: A brief review and postmortem diagnostic approach. Archives of Pathology & Laboratory Medicine. 2018 Jul;**142**(7):871-875. DOI: 10.5858/arpa.2017-0117-RS

[35] Zhibin Z, Peng S, Fang C. Fat embolism following a liposuction procedure. Neurology India. 2018;**66**(4):1206-1207. DOI: 10.4103/0028-3886.236965

[36] Franco FF, Tincani AJ, Meirelles LR, Kharmandayan P, Guidi MC. Occurrence of fat embolism after liposuction surgery with or without lipografting: An experimental study. Annals of Plastic Surgery. 2011;**67**(2):101-105. DOI: 10.1097/SAP.0b013e3181fe32b6

[37] You JS, Chung YE, Baek SE, Chung SP, Kim MJ. Imaging findings of liposuction with an emphasis on postsurgical complications. Korean Journal of Radiology. 2015;**16**(6):1197-1206. DOI: 10.3348/kjr.2015.16.6.1197

[38] Moura FC, Cunha LP, Monteiro ML. Bilateral visual loss after liposuction: Case report and review of the literature. Clinics (São Paulo, Brazil). 2006;**61**(5):489-491

[39] Ezzeddine H, Husari A, Nassar H, Kanso M, Nounou GE, Khalife M, et al. Life threatening complications post-liposuction. Aesthetic Plastic Surgery. 2018;**42**(2):384-387. DOI: 10.1007/s00266-017-1058-x

[40] Lehnhardt M, Homann HH, Daigeler A, Hauser J, Palka P, Steinau HU. Major and lethal complications of liposuction: A review of 72 cases in Germany between 1998 and 2002. Plastic and Reconstructive Surgery. 2008;**121**(6):396e-403e. DOI: 10.1097/PRS.0b013e318170817a

[41] Granados-Tinajero S, Buenrostro-Vásquez C, Buck-Soltero JA. Oxigenación hiperbárica. In: Anestesia en Sistema Respiratorio y Ventilación Mecánica. Editorial ILCSA, S.A. Mexico. 2013. pp. 569-589

[42] Granados-Tinajero S, Buenrostro C. Oxigenación hiperbárica en cirugía plástica reconstructiva. Anestesia en Mexico. 2009;**21**(1):35-43

[43] Buras JA, Stahl GL, Svoboda KK, Reenstra WR. Hyperbaric oxygen downregulates ICAM-1 expression induced by hypoxia and hypoglycemia: The role of NOS. American Journal of Physiology. Cell Physiology. 2000;**278**(2):C292-C302. DOI: 10.1152/ajpcell.2000.278.2.C292

[44] Tjärnström J, Holmdahl L, Falk P, Falkenberg M, Arnell P, Risberg B. Effects of hyperbaric oxygen on expression of fibrinolytic factors of human endothelium in a simulated ischaemia/reperfusion situation. Scandinavian Journal of Clinical and Laboratory Investigation. 2002;**61**(7):539-545. DOI: 10.1080/003655101753218300

Chapter 5

Regional Anesthesia for Urgent Reconstructive Surgery

Shivakumar M. Channabasappa

Additional information is available at the end of the chapter

http://dx.doi.org/10.5772/intechopen.80647

Abstract

In polytrauma patients, the primary goal is to administer early resuscitation and effective analgesia with medications or techniques, which minimally affect the patient's physiology. Adequate pain control will reduce posttraumatic stress disorder and facilitate in early functional recovery and better wound healing. Most of these polytrauma patients are hemodynamically unstable and require anesthesia and analgesia with techniques that produce minimum hemodynamic derangements; these techniques depend on the severity of trauma. The complexity of the surgery varies from primary closure to free flap reconstruction. More complicated injuries with larger tissue loss require free flap cover for better wound healing and optimal functional outcome. Optimum care of flap is an important part of perioperative management to prevent flap failure. Regional anesthesia has been proven to prevent flap failure by increasing perfusion to injured area by blocking local sympathetic system and minimizing pain-induced vasospasm. Postoperative prevention of hypothermia maintaining normocarbia plays a vital role in maintaining perfusion of free flap and prevention of flap failure. Regional anesthesia allows safe management of these patients.

Keywords: reconstructive surgery, regional anesthesia, trauma

1. Introduction

Anesthetic management of acutely injured patients scheduled for urgent reconstructive surgery is associated with multiple challenges. These patients are hemodynamically unstable requires early resuscitation, maintaining airway and providing effective analgesia is primary goal. In trauma patients, provision of adequate analgesia is usually delayed due to critical state of patients and adverse effects of systemic analgesics on different organs, with advent of newer technology and regional anesthesia can be effectively given to all trauma victims with minimum adverse events. Patients with polytrauma who needs emergency reconstructive surgery are associated with neurovascular injury, which requires early assessment and management which is altered by administration of narcotic based analgesics due to sedation and delirium associated with opioid analgesics.

Patients with polytrauma associated with an average of two fractures, and 5% of patients with more severe injuries are associated with five or more fractures. Most of these patients are associated with femoral fractures (16.5%) followed by tibia (12.6%) and clavicle (10.4%) fractures. The polytrauma patients who had fewer fractures are associated with severe traumatic brain injury (TBI) and lower Glasgow coma scale (GCS) and had increased in hospital mortality [1]. Since most of regional anesthesia (RA) procedures involve the extremities their role in anesthetic management for urgent reconstructive surgery seems well suited.

Polytrauma due to accident significantly activates stress hormones, inflammatory mediators and catabolism, from the time of injury extending through to rehabilitation. Pathophysiological changes after trauma may be increased by systemic opioids and other analgesics. Adverse effects of narcotic analgesics include drowsiness, respiratory depression vomiting, constipation deranged sleep and dependence [2].

Regional anesthesia in elective surgical procedure is widely used either alone or along with general anesthesia. RA has advantage of minimizing stress response to injury; these advantages are often not translated to the trauma patients. Early and late advantages of RA are often overlooked for fear of rare complications and less effective and more deleterious narcotic based analgesics predominate.

The benefit of peripheral nerve blocks (PNB) is the provision of high quality analgesia that is site specific and devoid of any systemic side effects. RA confers several other advantages over general anesthesia for trauma patient including reduction in opioid requirement and length of stay in emergency or critical care units, improved comfort and safety for transport, reduction in the stress response to injury. The capability of CPNB to provide long-term analgesia and surgical anesthesia during frequent trips to the operating room is a significant benefit of this pain management technique [3, 4].

Post traumatic patients are associated with posttraumatic stress disorder (PTSD) and chronic regional pain syndrome (CRPS) following acute injury, more than 75% of severe polytrauma patients develop chronic pain syndrome. Chronic pain syndrome is defined as pain persisting for more than 12 weeks following acute injury [5]. Development of chronic pain syndrome following acute injury is multifactorial. However, the risk factor that appears to be most predictive of eventual chronic pain is the intensity of acute pain at the time of injury. RA has been shown to significantly reduce acute pain intensity in traumatic injury. While it is attractive to assume that quality regional blockade early during an injury would prevent the development of chronic pain.

2. Rationale for regional anesthesia use in reconstructive surgery

Regional block offers many advantages of an ideal analgesic. Specific and unique advantages include superior analgesia, decreased postoperative delirium and psychosis, preserved sleep cycle, attenuation of stress response to injury, decreased nausea and vomiting, decreased posttraumatic chronic pain syndrome, and reduced systemic side-effects of opioids. Administration of regional anesthesia averts the risk of airway complications associated with airway instrumentation during general anesthesia and positive pressure ventilation, such as failure to secure airway, aspiration pneumonia and aggravation of cervical cord injury. Anesthesiologists encounter patients with critical trauma at various times during ongoing care, from prehospital resuscitation, stabilization in the emergency department, the management of the anesthesia and the intensive care unit, to the pain treatment service. Each stage offers the opportunity to provide regional anesthesia to trauma patients [6].

3. Key points for using regional anesthesia in reconstructive surgery

- Reconstructive surgery procedures rely on different approaches to local and regional anesthesia.
- Systemic toxicity associated local anesthetics during regional anesthesia and peripheral nerve block is a major anesthetic complication in poly-trauma patients due to rapid LA absorption into the vascular system.
- Less common complications associated with regional anesthesia are direct nerve injury, hematoma, pneumothorax, inadequate block, phrenic nerve palsy, Horner's syndrome and compartment syndrome.
- RA is ideal, site-specific and high-quality analgesia without risk of respiratory depression, drowsiness and bleeding associated with opioid and non-steroidal anti-inflammatory drugs.
- Increased availability of point of care ultrasound equipment and improved technology has made the administration of RA accurate, repeatable and with fewer complications.
- Regional anesthesia provides effective analgesia in critically ill trauma patients with multiple rib fractures, hip fractures and other injuries, where administration of systemic analgesics is associated with inadequate analgesia and delayed recovery.
- Compartment syndrome associated with RA and peripheral nerve blocks due to delay in diagnosis can be prevented by judicious use of low concentration local anesthetics and early mobilization.
- Decrease in the complications associated with RA due to advances in technology and better training. It can be administered outside the operating room to provide an arrival block with analgesia superior to the beginning of patient care.

4. Application of regional anesthesia in trauma management

4.1. Thoracoabdominal trauma

Thoracic injuries include: blunt chest injuries such as rib fractures, flail chest and pulmonary contusion are common, with significant morbidity and mortality. Pain impairs with adequate respiratory movements predisposing to atelectasis, pneumonia and retention of secretion. RA modalities include erector spinae plane block, serrates anterior plane blocks, cervical and thoracic epidural analgesia (TEA), intercostal blocks, paravertebral block and intrapleural catheters. Thoracotomy for acute chest injury is associated with excruciating postoperative pain which impairs with respiratory movement during postsurgical period, and it also associated with more than 50% chronic pain syndrome, which is debilitating. Cervical and thoracic epidural block is gold standard for managing postthoracotomy pain syndrome. Chest injury with multiple rib fractures are encountered in more than 10% of trauma patients, requiring adequate analgesia to prevent atelectasis, pulmonary infections. Thoracic paravertebral block and thoracic and cervical epidural analgesia provide excellent pain relief in these patients. However, previously reported reduction in duration of mechanical ventilation, hospital stay, and mortality rate are unequivocal [7]. Trauma patients are associated, with coagulopathy due to hemorrhage, massive blood transfusion or thromboprophylaxis and most of these patients are hypovolemic, which preclude the use thoracic epidural blocks.

4.1.1. *Thoracic paravertebral block*

Thoracic paravertebral block (TPVB) provides excellent unilateral analgesia in chest trauma patients. Segmental thoracic dermatomal block associated with less frequent hypotension in these hypovolemic patients as compared to TEA. TPVB may be administered in patients with anticoagulation, concomitant spinal injury, allowing adequate analgesia without interfering in neurological assessment [8].

4.1.2. *Intercostal nerve block (ICNB)*

Involves injection of local anesthetics around the posterior segment of intercostal nerves. Contrast studies of intercostal injections have demonstrated the spread of contrast media to adjacent dermatomes representing spread via the extra pleural or paravertebral spaces. ICNB can be used in minor chest injuries with unilateral less than three rib fractures but in major chest injuries and for thoracotomy, ICNB are less effective, these patients require more effective pain management modalities such as TPVB and TEA. Radiographic studies of intercostal injections have demonstrated the spread of injectate to adjacent dermatomes representing spread via extra pleural or paravertebral spaces [9].

4.1.3. *Intrapleural analgesia (IPA)*

Involves injection of a local anesthetic agent between parietal and visceral pleura through an indwelling catheter. This produces a multiple intercostal nerve block by gravity dependent diffusion of local anesthetic agent across the parietal pleura, producing unilateral analgesia at multiple dermatomal segments. Advantages of intrapleural blocks involve relatively easy technique, minimal hemodynamics derangements, no motor weakness and bowel and bladder involvement. This modality of analgesia can be used in blunt chest injury patients. IPA is associated with disadvantages like unpredictable analgesia, systemic local anesthetic toxicity, loss of local anesthetics through chest tube (loss of local anesthetics through chest tubes can be minimized by transient clamping of chest tubes). Other adverse effects of intra pleural block includes pneumothorax, hemothorax, and decreased diaphragmatic contractility due to disproportionate diffusion of LA and adversely affecting its function [10].

4.1.4. *Abdominal plane blocks*

The transverse abdominal plane (TAP) block and rectus sheath block provide somatic sensory analgesia to the anterior abdominal wall. The anterior divisions of the spinal nerves T7-L1 cross between the internal oblique and the transversus abdominis muscles, and they perforate the rectus abdominis muscle. These nerves can be blocked injecting local anesthetics between internal oblique and transversus abdominis muscles (TAP), or between rectus sheath and rectus muscle (rectus sheath block). Although these blocks are widely used for postoperative analgesia, its use in trauma patients is limited. Recent data suggest that erector spinae plane block or quadratus lumborum block may be more useful abdominal trauma and pelvic fractures.

4.2. Limb trauma

Upper limb injuries are particularly suited to peripheral nerve blocks for prolonged pain management and repeated surgical interventions. Brachial plexus block (BPB) provides superior analgesia, reduced narcotic consumption and shorter hospital stay compared with general anesthesia for ambulatory upper limb trauma surgery. For bilateral upper limb injuries ultrasound guided BPB with distal approaches and peripheral nerve blocks are recommended to minimize local anesthetic toxicity and risk of diaphragmatic palsy and respiratory distress.

Options for pain management in upper limb include the following:

- Brachial plexus block (e.g. interscalene, supraclavicular, infra-clavicular and axillary approaches)
- Peripheral nerve block (e.g. radial, median, and ulnar)
- Intravenous regional anesthesia (IVRA)

4.2.1. *Lower limb trauma*

Regional anesthesia for managing patients with polytrauma challenging, appropriate use of regional anesthesia can complement ATLS management priorities. Peripheral nerve blocks are generally safer and more practical than neuraxial techniques in hemodynamically unstable trauma patients. The challenge of translating benefit from regional blocks to patient care pathway requires appropriate infrastructure and training. Regional block provides main attributes of an ideal analgesic. Advantages of RA include superior analgesia, attenuation of stress response decreased postoperative delirium and avoidance of systemic side-effects.

Regional anesthesia and peripheral nerve blocks are increasingly used for lower limb trauma. Advances in ultrasonography in regional anesthesia increases the percentage of block success and reduces the requirement of local anesthetics. Femoral and lumbar plexus blocks for femur fractures are effective and safe in hemodynamically unstable and elderly trauma patients.

Regional anesthesia for hip fractures is associated with less delirium and better analgesia. For lower leg injuries, sciatic nerve block by parasacral, mid sciatic or popliteal approach facilitate superior analgesia. Ankle blocks are almost replaced by popliteal nerve block with saphenous nerve block to allow surgery to the foot.

Options for pain management in lower limb include the following:

- Lumbar epidural
- Subarachnoid block
- Lumbar/sacral plexus block
- Compartment blocks (e.g. fascia iliac)
- Peripheral nerves (e.g. femoral sciatic, saphenous, and obturator)

5. Limitations of regional anesthesia in trauma

Careful risk–benefit analysis must be used while considering RA techniques. Circumstances where RA is not appropriate include: the debate on whether peripheral blocks are safer when performed on awake or anesthetized patients is unresolved. Available evidence is low-level and conflicting and expert opinion is divergent. Regional anesthesia in sedated patients hide presentation of complications associated with RA like intraneural injections and local anesthetic toxicity.

Regional anesthesia is contraindicated in the following situations:

- Trauma victims with hemorrhagic shock and threatened airway
- Traumatic brain injury
- Raised intracranial pressure (for neuraxial blocks)
- Coagulopathy
- Patient refusal for regional anesthesia
- Allergy to LA
- Lack of appropriate training, equipment, and care bundles

6. Special problems

6.1. Compartment syndrome

Compartment syndrome is the most dreaded complication following a limb trauma. Acute compartment syndrome commonly occurs following forearm and leg fractures in young adults less than 35 years of age. Who has more tissue mass. Acute trauma leads edema of injured tissues, due to closed osteofacial compartment in forearm and leg, increased pressure following tissue swelling causes collapse of arterioles and capillaries, which leads to cessation of circulation and tissue hypoxia. Following tissue hypoxia inflammatory mediators will be released leading to increased vascular permeability and worsening tissue edema. Regional anesthesia and peripheral nerve blocks provide excellent perioperative analgesia, but few clinicians fear an anesthetized limb may delay the diagnosis of acute compartment syndrome by masking symptoms due to regional block. However, sensitivity of these subjective symptoms is less than 20% [11, 12].

There are only five case reports of compartment syndrome following peripheral nerve blocks. At present, it is difficult to make direct correlation peripheral nerve blocks to compartment syndrome. The use of lower concentration of local anesthetics, intermittent analgesic, measuring compartment pressure in high-risk patients, limb elevation and careful monitoring are key for early diagnosis and prompt treatment.

6.2. Preexisting nerve injury

The "double crush syndrome" proposes that patients with pre-existing nerve lesions are more susceptible to further injury when exposed to a secondary insult. Preexisting nerve injury in trauma victims may be exacerbated by nerve blocks, either by direct damaging nerve or due to local anesthetic induced neuronal toxicity, although the evidence of neuronal injury due to PNB is unequivocal.

Careful neurological assessment risk stratification and usage of ultrasonography for peripheral nerve blocks will substantially reduce direct nerve injury. Usage of USG during peripheral nerve blocks allows low volume and concentration of LA by precisely localizing neuronal structures, and this reduces the incidence of neuronal injury [13].

6.3. Anticoagulation

Trauma victims with multiple injuries predisposes to coagulopathy, this may be exacerbated by massive blood transfusion, hypothermia, medications and disseminated intravascular coagulation. Risk depends on the patient, mechanism of injury and medicines. In acute phase hypothermia and hemorrhage may lead to a coagulopathy. Best way is to individually weigh risk against the benefit of RA in trauma patients with coagulation abnormalities [14]. If the RA is chosen for the patients with coagulation abnormalities, extreme vigilance and monitoring for eventual side effects is mandatory.

Recommendations for performing RA should be done according to latest American Society of Regional Anesthesia and Pain Medicine guidelines [15]. Spinal and epidural anesthesia in patients the coagulopathy poses greater risk than peripheral nerve blocks since hemorrhage into the central neuraxis causes more disastrous complication. Thromboprophylaxis in trauma victims could contraindicate usage of neuraxial block. Choosing appropriate anticoagulation schedules and usage of ultrasonography for regional anesthesia provides the safer option in anticoagulated patients.

Recent advances in point-of-care coagulation testing like thromboelastography provide rapid, objective assessment of hemostatic function. This may be used before interventions, to detect type of coagulopathy and to administer specific coagulation factors.

6.4. Chronic pain

Chronic pain is more common following trauma than often realized, inadequate management of acute pain increases the risk of development of chronic pain syndrome. It may be due to nociceptive pain or often include a neuropathic component, which can be difficult to treat. There are several pain syndromes such as complex regional pain syndrome (CRPS), postamputation pain, and posttraumatic stress disorder which are specifically associated with trauma.

Early, effective and sustained analgesia and usage of peripheral nerve blocks after injury decreases the incidence and severity of chronic pain syndromes. Administration of low and therapeutic doses of antidepressants, oral ketamine and gabapentin should be considered for persistent pain [16, 17].

7. Conclusion

Trauma represents a considerable and increasing demand on healthcare resources. Early resuscitation and on-arrival block forms primary goal initial management of polytrauma patients. Advances in regional anesthesia, better training and availability of point of care sonography allowed safer administration of RA and peripheral nerve block in critically ill polytrauma patients. Early administration of peripheral nerve blocks minimizes pulmonary and cardiovascular complications, decreases incidence of posttraumatic stress disorder and chronic pain syndrome, allows prompt mobilization and significantly reduces consumption of narcotic analgesics. Careful use of regional anesthetics in polytrauma patients, reduce duration of hospital stay and delirium in elderly patients. Regional anesthesia and peripheral nerve blocks are not devoid of adverse effects like systemic LA toxicity, neurovascular injury, and compartment syndrome. Selecting proper regional anesthesia technique, usage of appropriate local anesthetic concentration and volume, these complications can be reduced. RA is more versatile and reliable than ever before, with appropriate patient selection and usage of ultrasonography, such interventions are effective and safe. When used carefully in selected polytrauma patients regional anesthesia provides a cost-effective and safer method of analgesia in injured patients in both during surgery and perioperative settings.

Conflict of interest

Nil.

Thanks

I would like to thank my wife Dr. Shruthi for her support in preparing this chapter.

Author details

Shivakumar M. Channabasappa

Address all correspondence to: drshivakumar.m.c@gmail.com

Department of Anesthesiology and Critical Care, Subbaiah Institute of Medical Sciences, Shimoga, Karnataka, India

References

[1] Banerjee M, Bouillon B, Shafizadeh S, Paffrath T, Lefering R, Wafaisade A, German Trauma Registry Group. Epidemiology of extremity injuries in multiple trauma patients. Injury. 2013;**44**(8):1015-1021. DOI: 10.1016/j.injury.2012.12.007

[2] Fleming I, Egeler C. Regional anaesthesia for trauma: An update. Continuing Education in Anaesthesia Critical Care & Pain. 2014;**14**(3):136-141. DOI: https://doi.org/10.1093/bjaceaccp/mkt048

[3] Buckenmaier CC, McKnight GM, Winkley JV, Bleckner LL, Shannon C, Klein SM, Lyons RC, Chiles JH. Continuous peripheral nerve block for battlefield anesthesia and evacuation. Regional Anesthesia and Pain Medicine. 2005;**30**(2):202-205

[4] Plunkett AR, Brown DS, Rogers JM, Buckenmaier CC 3rd. Supraclavicular continuous peripheral nerve block in a wounded soldier: When ultrasound is the only option. British Journal of Anaesthesia. 2006;**97**(5):715-717. DOI: 10.1093/bja/ael218

[5] Radresa O, Chauny JM, Lavigne G, Piette E, Paquet J, Daoust R. Current views on acute to chronic pain transition in post-traumatic patients: Risk factors and potential for pre-emptive treatments. Journal of Trauma and Acute Care Surgery. 2014;**76**(4):1142-1150. DOI: 10.1097/TA.0000000000000188

[6] Berben SA, Meijs TH, van Dongen RT, van Vugt AB, Vloet LC, Mintjes-de Groot JJ, van Achterberg T. Pain prevalence and pain relief in trauma patients in the accident & emergency department. Injury. 2008;**39**(5):578-585. DOI: 10.1016/j.injury.2007.04.013

[7] Carrier FM, Turgeon AF, Nicole PC, Trépanier CA, Fergusson DA, Thauvette D, Lessard MR. Effect of epidural analgesia in patients with traumatic rib fractures: A systematic review and meta-analysis of randomized controlled trials. Canadian Journal of Anaesthesia. 2009;**56**(3):230-242. DOI: 10.1007/s12630-009-9052-7

[8] Karmakar MK, Chui PT, Joynt GM, Ho AM. Thoracic paravertebral block for management of pain associated with multiple fractured ribs in patients with concomitant lumbar spinal trauma. Regional Anesthesia and Pain Medicine. 2001;**26**(2):169-173. DOI: 10.1053/rapm.2001.21086

[9] Hwang EG, Lee Y. Effectiveness of intercostal nerve block for management of pain in rib fracture patients. Journal of Exercise Rehabilitation. 2014;**10**(4):241-244. DOI: 10.12965/jer.140137

[10] Simon BJ, Cushman J, Barraco R, Lane V, Luchette FA, Miglietta M, Roccaforte DJ, Spector R, EAST Practice Management Guidelines Work Group. Pain management guidelines for blunt thoracic trauma. The Journal of Trauma. 2005;**59**(5):1256-1267

[11] Ulmer T. The clinical diagnosis of compartment syndrome of the lower leg: Are clinical findings predictive of the disorder? Journal of Orthopaedic Trauma. 2002;**16**(8):572-577

[12] Mar GJ, Barrington MJ, McGuirk BR. Acute compartment syndrome of the lower limb and the effect of postoperative analgesia on diagnosis. British Journal of Anaesthesia. 2009;**102**(1):3-11. DOI: 10.1093/bja/aen330

[13] Neal JM, Barrington MJ, Brull R, Hadzic A, Hebl JR, Horlocker TT, Huntoon MA, Kopp SL, Rathmell JP, Watson JC. The second ASRA practice advisory on neurologic complications associated with regional anesthesia and pain medicine: Executive Summary 2015. Regional Anesthesia and Pain Medicine. 2015;**40**(5):401-430. DOI: 10.1097/AAP.0000000000000286

[14] Horlocker TT, Wedel DJ, Rowlingson JC, Enneking FK, Kopp SL, Benzon HT, Brown DL, Heit JA, Mulroy MF, Rosenquist RW, Tryba M, Yuan CS. Regional anesthesia in the patient receiving antithrombotic or thrombolytic therapy: American Society of Regional Anesthesia and Pain Medicine Evidence-Based Guidelines (third edition). Regional Anesthesia and Pain Medicine. 2010;**35**(1):64-101

[15] Horlocker TT, Wedel DJ, Rowlingson JC, Enneking FK. Executive summary: Regional anesthesia in the patient receiving antithrombotic or thrombolytic therapy: American Society of Regional Anesthesia and Pain Medicine Evidence-Based Guidelines (third edition). Regional Anesthesia and Pain Medicine. 2010;**35**(1):102-105. DOI: 10.1097/AAP.0b013e3181c15dd0

[16] Bajwa ZH, Simopoulos TT, Pal J, Kraemer JJ, Chopra P, Nagda JV, Najib U, Celestin J, Sial K, Ahmad B, Warfield C, Steinman TI, Wootton J. Low and therapeutic doses of antidepressants are associated with similar response in the context of multimodal treatment of pain. Pain Physician. 2009;**12**(5):893-900

[17] Blonk MI, Koder BG, van den Bemt PM, Huygen FJ. Use of oral ketamine in chronic pain management: A review. European Journal of Pain. 2010;**14**(5):466-472. DOI: 10.1016/j.ejpain.2009.09.005

Chapter 6

Pain Management in Plastic Surgery

I Gusti Ngurah Mahaalit Aribawa, Made Wiryana,
Tjokorda Gde Agung Senapathi and
Pontisomaya Parami

Additional information is available at the end of the chapter

http://dx.doi.org/10.5772/intechopen.79302

Abstract

Most patients who undergo cosmetic surgery do not report pain during the immediate postoperative period. However, most patients who underwent liposuction combined with or without other plastic surgical procedure suffer pain after surgery. There are three main techniques in acute pain management postoperatively which are systemic analgesia, regional analgesia, and local/topical analgesia, and these are the extent of trauma during the procedure, surgeon's skill, prior disease, location and type of incision, and psychological and cultural factors. Treatment for each type of plastic surgery and the resulting pain require techniques that can be used as single method or combined with each other to relieve postoperative pain after plastic surgery. Nausea, vomiting, constipation, somnolence, etc., are well-known adverse effects of opioids. Although these effects may seem minor, they can lead to significant complications following some type of plastic surgeries, for example, face-lift hematoma following nausea and vomiting, pulmonary complications from respiratory depression, and even thromboembolic phenomena from bed rest following prolonged opioid use. Multimodal pain management has been documented to increase patient satisfaction and reduce both opioid use and the incidence of PONV. Combination of pain management in plastic surgery included patient-controlled analgesia intravenous (PCA-IV), patient-controlled epidural analgesia (PCEA), patient-controlled regional analgesia (PCRA), field block (TAP block), continuous wound infusion system using pain pump and tumescent analgesia with local anesthetics.

Keywords: postoperative pain, IV-PCA, PCEA, PCRA, field block, TAP block, tumescent analgesia, opioids, NSAIDs

1. Introduction

Plastic surgery has become increasingly done over the last decades. The surgeon and patients become aware of the importance of postoperative pain control. This has occurred in part in an attempt to improve the patient experience and satisfaction. However, pain remains a major patient concern. Most patients who undergo cosmetic surgery do not report pain during the immediate postoperative period. However, most patients who underwent liposuction combined with or without other surgical procedure report pain after surgery. Pain is unpleasant sensory and emotional experience associated with tissue injury [2]. Postoperative pain is mainly derived from acute tissue manipulation during the surgical procedure. In fact, a recent study documented that 30–80% of patients undergoing outpatient surgery encountered moderate-to-severe postoperative pain. The characteristics of pain that should be evaluated are onset, location, irradiation, type of pain, duration, and pain-related behavioral responses [2–4].

Along with this increased awareness of the importance for pain management, a variety of newer analgesics modalities designed to reduce pain have arrived on the scene. In the era of health care reformation, it is important to consider that pain management techniques can contribute to the overall value of care that is delivered to patients.

1.1. Concept of multimodal pain management

Treatment for each type of plastic surgery and resulted pain requires a specific approach and must be individualized to the patient. There are three main techniques for acute postoperative pain management: systemic analgesia, regional analgesia, and local/topical analgesia. Systemic analgesia can be given through intravenous injection, oral or rectal route, intramuscular, and skin patch. Regional analgesia technique can be divided into neuraxial analgesia and peripheral nerve block. Currently, pain management through intravenous injection or continuous neuraxial and peripheral nerve blocks is more controllable and safer since the invention of pain pump, which commonly use the principal of patient-controlled analgesia. Opioids, nonsteroidal anti-inflammatory drugs (NSAIDs), mild analgesics, local anesthetics, etc., are all valuable in the multimodal pain management [4–6].

Nausea, vomiting, constipation, somnolence, etc., are well-known adverse effects of opioids. Although these effects may seem minor to some, they can lead to significant complications following certain types of plastic surgery, for example, face-lift hematoma following nausea and vomiting, pulmonary complications from respiratory depression, and even thromboembolic phenomena from bed rest following prolonged opioid use. In fact, a recent study documented adverse side effects in 17% of patients due to opioids. Most importantly, multimodal pain therapy including pharmaceutical agents mentioned above, long-acting local anesthetic preparations, and pain pumps may in large part replace isolated narcotic treatment of postoperative pain. This approach has been documented to increase patient satisfaction and reduce both opioid use and the incidence of nausea and vomiting in a large variety of nonfacial esthetic procedures. Although this multimodal treatment seems to have significant benefits, postoperative dosing becomes more complex, and adverse drug interactions and drug overdose become more likely [1–10].

There are some combinations that is proven to have a good effect in multimodal analgesia, such as paracetamol and NSAIDs, paracetamol with opioids, nonselective NSAIDs or selective cyclooxygenase (COX)-2 inhibitors with opioids, and alpha-2-delta modulators (gabapentin and pregabalin) with opioids, N-methyl-D-aspartate (NMDA) antagonists ketamine and magnesium, also alpha-2-agonists clonidine and dexmedetomidine with opioids. Combination of central neuraxial analgesia through epidural with NSAIDs proved favorable by suppressing stress response and suppressing pro-inflammatory factor [4–9].

2. Systemic analgesia

There are several systemic analgesic protocols to relieve postoperative pain in plastic surgery, but the IV administration of opioid and nonopioid analgesics is the most used. In the following paragraphs, each one of these managements is described, being possible for the combination of the different alternatives of analgesia.

2.1. Oral administration

Postoperative pain management for ambulatory patients usually is treated with NSAIDs. This type of analgesics is the most important treatment for nociceptive pain. These kind of patients may also need a short-acting opioids such as hydrocodone, oxycodone, and acetaminophen. In immediate postoperative pain management, we prefer to use short-acting opioids rather than long-acting ones. However, if the patient is already on long-acting opioid before surgery, it is more appropriate to continue the long-acting opioid with combination of short-acting opioid for postoperative pain [3–9].

2.2. Intravenous bolus injection

Intravenous (IV) injection drugs that are commonly used as postoperative pain management are opioids (morphine and oxycodone). They are given based on patient's need, usually for every 2–4 h. This condition can become a burden for both nurse and patient when the ratio between nurse and patient is low. NSAIDs also can be given intravenously for a short period, 1–2 days [5, 7, 9, 11–13].

2.3. Intravenous patient-controlled analgesia (PCA-IV)

Patient-controlled analgesia (PCA) was used since 1971. PCA is one of the pain management techniques using a programmable pump intravenous device. The machine is put at patient's bedside and connected to the IV line than contains a bag of premixed opioid solution. The patient can self-administer analgesic on demand by pressing the button connected to the PCA machine. The demand dose is already determined by the physician. The machine will lock for the amount of time before it can send another demand dose (lockout period), so it can protect the patient from overdosing. PCA device can also release the drug at a low-dose continuous infusion rate [3]. There are several advantages of PCA such as painless route to deliver opioid, give accurate analgesia, help the nursing staff in patient's pain control, and ensure the medication level compared with intermittent bolus injection or continuous IV infusion of opioid. PCA is used when the patient cannot take oral medication either in preoperative or postoperative time or has nausea that causing the patient unable to take oral medication. PCA often use to control severe pain level such as burn injuries.

Minimal analgesia can be reached with opioid titration until minimum effective analgesia concentration (MEAC) can be reached, which becomes the border between pain and analgesia. Furthermore, the dosage for causing analgesia varied among the patients and can be concluded that variability in opioid's pharmacodynamic causes differences in the dosage. Individual MEAC can be determined by level of opioid endogen in preoperative cerebrospinal fluid. Patient with higher level of opioid endogen in cerebrospinal fluid needs lower MEAC to achieve and maintain the analgesia effect [3, 5, 7, 9, 11–15] (**Figure 1**).

In the figure above, X axis is the opioid plasma concentration and Y axis is the pain intensity from severe pain to no pain. Small circles show correlation between opioid concentration and pain intensity in an interval of increased opioid concentration. At the beginning, progressive increase of opioid concentration does not change pain intensity, but then with a little increase of opioid concentration, it can decrease pain intensity until pain is resolved. Increase of opioid concentration after this point will not give an extra effect.

2.3.1. *PCA variable*

PCA can be given in many methods, and the following two are the most common methods used in daily practice:

- Demand dose (the dosage has been made by the anesthetist and given by patient to him/herself in a given period of time)
- Continuous infusion/background infusion along with demand dose in accordance with patient's need.

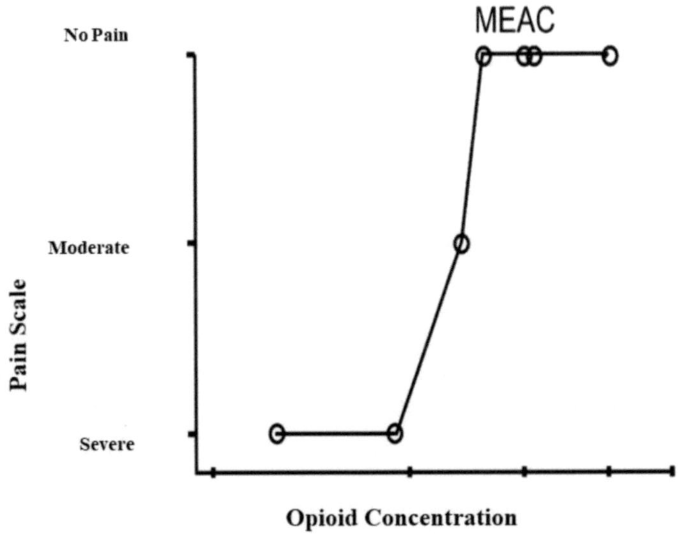

Figure 1. Response to opioid concentration and pain intensity [17].

2.3.1.1. Programmed intermittent bolus (PIB)

PIB is a specific dosage of drug that is programmed in PCA to give automatic bolus drug in specific intervals. PIB does not depend on demand dose or continuous infusion. PIB is usually used for epidural analgesia or peripheral nerve block analgesia. Time interval is around 15–60 min, which means every for 15–60 min. PCA machine will automatically give bolus drug in a specific dose. For all PCA method, there are basic variables, such as: (a) initial bolus dose, (b) demand dose, (c) lockout interval, (d) Background infusion, (e) Maximum dose limitation 1 and 4 h [15–19].

2.3.1.2. Initial bolus dose

It is possible to give drugs titration when activated by the program (not the patient). Initial bolus dose can be used by the nurse in postanesthesia care unit (PACU) to titrate opioid dose until reach MEAC or by the nurse at ward to administer the extra dose for the breakthrough pain. Initial bolus dose is the key for the success in pain management using PCA. Without it, there is a big possibility that pain may not be resolve adequately and patient can be disappointed using the PCA machine [15–19].

2.3.1.3. Demand dose

Demand dose is also known as incremental dose or PCA dose. It is amount of analgesia that is given to the patient when patient press the demand button. PCA dose aims to maintain opioid level in MEAC level. PCA dose is the maintenance dose [15–19].

2.3.1.4. Lockout interval

To prevent opioid overdose with continuous demand, all PCA machines use lockout interval. It gives time lapse after administration of demand dose, and the machine will not respond to any demand dose, even though patient press the button, until certain time. This is one of the security systems in the PCA machine [15–19].

2.3.1.5. Background infusion

Infusion with constant speed is given without considering the patient's demand. Background infusion is seldom used for patients with acute pain because of risk of overdose. Background infusion is usually administered to the patients who use opioid with large dose previously. Background infusion can be given by electrical PCA machine. Continuous infusion used as adjuvant in administration of bolus dose can increase analgesia effect for the patient, so they can sleep without any disturbance due to pain. Disadvantages from this system are that opioid could still be given without considering the sedation level and can increase the risk of respiratory depression. Routine use of background infusion is not recommended. Background infusion may be useful in patients who are tolerant toward opioid, patients who are common in using opioid and need higher dose, or patients who have sleep disturbance at night due to pain [15–19].

2.3.1.6. Maximum dose limitation

Some machine may have time limit 1 or 4 h. This program limits patient interval either 1 or 4 h to get total cumulative dose. Usage of the interval 1 or 4 h is controversial. Prolimitation said that the limitation could give better security, while the contra side said there is no evidence that shows this limitation could give better security. In the other hand, if patient needs demand dose or PCA dose in large amount until it reaches the limitation for 1 or 4 h, may be they really need that much dose to resolve the pain; thus, it is not necessary to reach that need. The usual maximum dose for morphine is 10 mg in 1 h or 30 mg in 4 h. Keep in mind that PCA is used as maintenance therapies and pain should be under controlled before PCA is started. Disadvantages of this system are that opioid could still be given without considering the sedation level and can increase the risk of respiratory depression [15–19] (**Figure 2**).

2.4. Opioid for IV-PCA

Knowledge about pharmacology is the basic to use PCA effectively. A physician should understand not only indication and contraindication, but also pharmacodynamic and pharmacokinetic of opioid, including absorption, distribution, biotransformation, and elimination from many types of opioid. Besides that, a doctor needs to understand specific physiologic response that can be happened when a drug binds to specific receptor inside or outside the

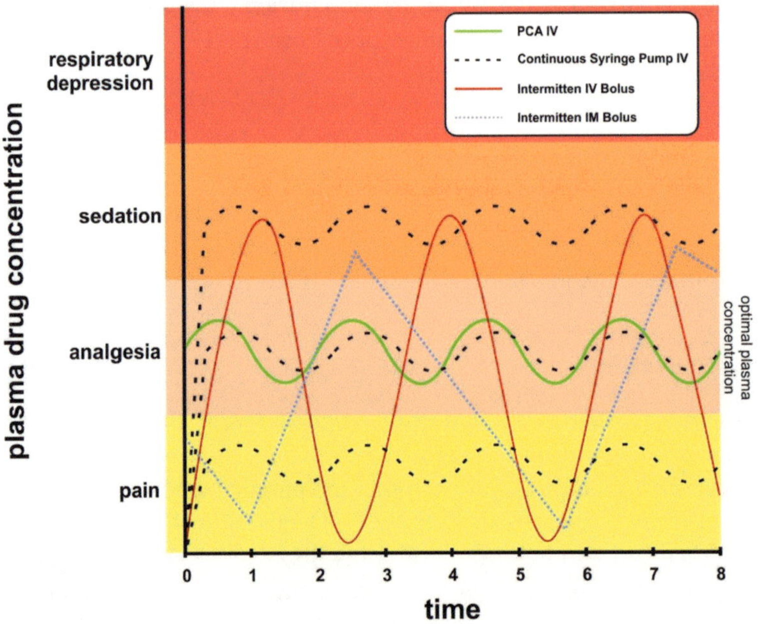

Figure 2. Comparison between plasma drug concentration and their administration. Plasma drug concentration after small frequent dose PCA administration compared with large dose intramuscular or intravenous administration every 2-4 hours and continuous infusion intravenous. Ideally, plasma drug concentration is constant in analgesia range without any surge of plasma drug concentration that lead to over sedation and respiratory depression or low level of drugs that cause inadequate analgesia. Small but frequent dose could be reached by PCA.

brain. Knowledge about all of the above will become essential to choose the right opioid that can be used in the PCA system. Parenteral opioid has three characters when binding with micro-opioid pure agonist, agonist-antagonist, and partial agonist. Character of pure agonist is the mainstay in acute pain management because can give full binding to microreceptor, and there is no maximal limit of analgesia (more opioid titration will give better effect in resolving pain.) However, there is a clinical maximal limitation that can give adverse effects such as sedation, respiratory depression, and often limit extra dose before reaching adequate level of analgesia. microagonist opioids are also effective in equianalgesic dose (i.e., 10 mg morphine = 2 mg hydromorphone = 100 mg meperidine) [15–19].

There are no significant differences in adverse effects due to opioids, even though patient can develop nausea, vomiting, or pruritus with one opioid, but not with other opioid drugs. All μ agonist decrease intestine movement, that contribute in ileus paralytic after surgery [15, 16, 18, 20].

Agonist-antagonist opioids activate κ receptor and antagonist toward microreceptor. Even though they are used with maximal effect limitation toward respiratory depression, it can give a wider safety margin, and this effect can happen with very large dose comparing it with microagonist. The most important thing is that agonist-antagonist has maximal limit of analgesic effect, so this group cannot make better analgesia compared with microagonist. Furthermore, agonist-antagonist drugs will induce acute withdrawal response in patients who receive microagonist opioids before. Due to activation of σ receptor, this group often induces psychotomimetic adverse effects. These type of opioids are uncommon to be used in PCA IV [15, 17, 18].

All opioids have been used successfully for PCA intravenous analgesia, with morphine as the most substance to be studied. Whatever opioid is chosen for intravenous PCA, knowledge about pharmacology is needed to control variable dose in PCA machine. Key component for effective PCA therapy is the right titration to get analgesia. Loading dose of morphine is 2–4 mg (or equianalgesic dose for alternative opioid) given every 5–10 min in postanesthesia care unit (PACU) until pain score ≤4 from 10 or if respiratory rate <12 times per minute, which will give limitation for the next opioid administration. It should become a consideration to use multimodal therapy to achieve optimal analgesia and to decrease the use of opioid and will decrease the possibility of adverse effect and respiratory depression (**Table 1**).

Opioid	Concentration	Demand dose	Lockout (min)	Continuous basal
Morphine	1 mg/ml	1–2 mg	6–10	0–2 mg/h
Fentanyl	10–20 μg/ml	20–50 μg	5–10	0–60 μg/h
Sufentanil	1–4 μg/ml	4–6 μg	1–10	0–8 μg/h
Hydromorphone	0.1–0.2 mg/ml	0.2–0.4	6–10	0–0.4 mg/h
Tramadol	10–20 mg/ml	10–20 mg	6–10	0–20 mg/h
Oxycodone	1–2 mg/ml	1–2 mg	5–10	0–2 mg/h

Continuous infusion is not recommended in early design.

Table 1. Common PCA regimen.

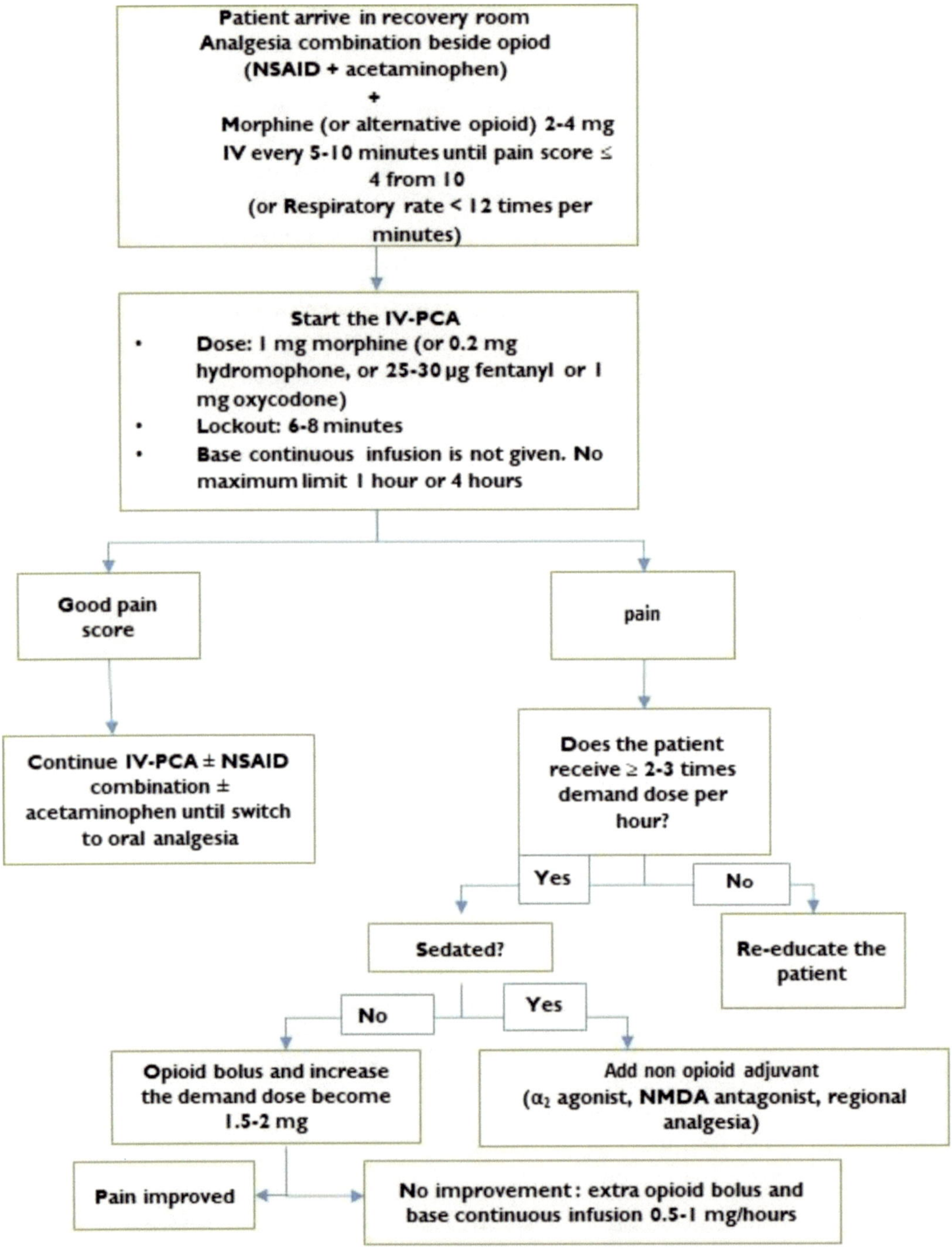

Figure 3. Simplified algorithm of IV-PCA management for basic setting of IV-PCA with morphine.

2.4.1. *Initial dose and adjusted dose*

There is no ideal dose in IV-PCA. Deciding dose for PCA depends on patient and expected postoperative pain. The key component of effective PCA therapy is initial titration to achieve pain-free condition or minimal pain before starting the IV-PCA program. One consideration is that multimodal therapy approach must start early to optimize the analgesia and decrease the need of opioid, so can decrease the adverse effect and respiratory depression. Pain management with PCA will fail if initial analgesia cannot be achieved. This condition will disappoint the patient who still feels pain even though the machine has been started. Patient will be frustrated and refuse to use PCA. Keep in mind that basic principle of PCA is to maintain the analgesia in optimal range for the patient [15, 17, 18] (**Figure 3**).

3. Regional analgesia

Analgesia with regional techniques has been fashionable due to its advantages: effective, safe, economical, and easy to perform. There are numerous techniques of perioperative analgesic blocks, which have benefited with the advent of ultrasound. The following paragraphs describe some procedures.

3.1. Central neuraxial analgesia

3.1.1. *Patient-controlled epidural analgesia (PCEA)*

Epidural analgesia is a safe and effective method to handle pain in any patient. It can be used for babies, children, adult, elderly in a short period (hours until days) or long period (weeks until months). Epidural analgesia can give superior regional analgesia compared with conventional systemic route (IV or oral) with minimum systemic side effect (nausea, sedation, or constipation). Drugs in epidural space are distributed through three main routes: (1) diffusion process through dura to cerebrospinal fluid, then to spinal cord or nerve root, (2) through uptake in epidural space blood vessel into systemic circulation, and (3) fat uptake of drug in epidural space where it can enter cerebrospinal fluid or systemic circulation. Epidural analgesia insertion can be combined with PCA machine to reduce pain with patient as the controller, which is known as patient-controlled epidural analgesia (PCEA). PCEA is an effective method to control pain with analgesia and local anesthesia through a catheter inside the epidural space connected with a pain pump that delivers small dose of drugs directly to the epidural space. Unlike systemic administration, drugs that are injected into the epidural space are potent because it is close to the opioid and alpha agonist receptors in dorsal horn. Due to small dose, the side effects are minimum such as nausea, sedation, and respiratory depression. Usage of this method is usually seen in obstetric surgery and postsurgery pain management for lower abdomen, thoracic, and cancer pain or chronic pain management. Currently, there are two main methods in PCEA usage such as demand dose only (PCEA dose) and continuous infusion with demand dose (PCEA + continuous infusion). Continuous infusion is an administration of drug with constant speed, without any consideration of patient's need. When the pain increases for some reason, activation of demand dose will cause administration of extra small dose that increases the drug's volume and the patient will be pain free. Some of PCEA machines make it possible for doctor to set other parameters in administration of drugs that is known as programmed intermittent epidural bolus (PIEB) [21–28] (**Table 2**).

Best pain management using epidural analgesia can be reached with combination of local anesthetic and opioid because they can work synergistic to decrease pain with fewer side effects than with single drug. All drugs and fluid that are injected into the epidural space should be free from preservative to avoid central nervous system toxicity [6].

The American Society of Anesthesiologist (ASA) published a clinical practice guidance to prevent infection from epidural analgesia. They recommend insertion of epidural catheter with aseptic technique, such as washing hand, sterile gloves, sterile gown, mask (used to cover mouth and nose), skin preparation, and sterile drapes around injection site. The tip of the epidural catheter should be placed based on the surgical dermatomes. Catheter should be fixed to minimize possibility of catheter misplace outside from the epidural space, migrate to subarachnoid space, or even migrate to a blood vessel. Dressing is adjusted so it will not cover the insertion. Nosocomial infection should be considered, and the use of prophylactics antibiotics is recommended, especially for patients with risk of infection (i.e., diabetics, patient who received steroid therapy or immunosuppression and patient who are hospitalized more than 48 h with epidural catheter) [29] (**Tables 3** and **4**).

Before PCEA is started, a loading dose should be administered to reach the initial block level using higher concentration of local anesthetic than the concentration in PCEA solution. Continuous rate for adult patients needs adjustment depending on patient's need. Continuous infusion is usually not used in PCEA [21–27] (**Table 5**).

3.2. Peripheral nerve blocks

Nerve block with local anesthetic in a specific location at or around the main nerve will depolarize the nerve and obtund the pain sensation in that specific area. Advantages of nerve block such as single accurate injection can block larger area of sensation without tissue distortion at the operative site. In the other hand, this method has the disadvantage of the sensation of

Surgery site and injury	**Epidural insertion**
Thoracic	T4-T8
Upper abdomen	T7-T10
Lower abdomen	T9-L1
Hip and lower extremities	L1-L4

Table 2. Epidural insertion based on surgery site.

Opioid	Concentration	Loading dose*	PCEA dose*	Lockout interval (min)	Continuous rate*	4 h limitation (ml)
Morphine	50 μg/ml	2–4 mg	2–4 ml	10–15	6–12 ml/h	40–70
Hydromorphone	10 μg/ml	500–1500 μg	2–4 ml	6–10	6–12 ml/h	40–70
Fentanyl	2–5 μg/ml	75–100 μg	2–4 ml	6	6–15 ml/h	40–70
Sufentanil	2 μg/ml	0.5 μg/kg	2–4 ml	6	0.1 μg/kg/h	40–70

*Depend on epidural catheter insertion, surgery condition, and patient's physical status.

Table 3. Opioid dose of PCEA guideline.

Incision site	Analgesia solution	Continuous infusion (ml/h)	Demand dose (ml)	Lockout interval (min)	PIEB (ml every)	
					Volume (ml)	Time (min)
Common Regimen	0.05% bupivacaine + 2–5 μg/ml fentanyl	4–10	2–6	10–15	—	—
	0.0625% bupivacaine + 2–5 μg/ml fentanyl	4–10	3–5	10–15	6–10	30–60
	0.1% bupivacaine +2–5 μg/ml fentanyl	6–8	2–3	10–20	10	60
	0.125% bupivacaine + 0.05–0.1 mg/ml morphine	4–6	5–10	15–20	—	—
	0.0625–0.125% levobupivacaine + sufentanil 0.5 μg /ml	10	5	10–15	10	60
	0.1% levobupivacaine + fentanyl 2 μg/ml	10	5	10–15	5–10	30–60
	0.1–0.2% ropivacaine + 2–5 μg/ml fentanyl	3–5	2–5	10–20	5 2.5	30 15
Thoracic	0.0625–0.125% bupivacaine + 2–5 μg/ml fentanyl	3–4	2–3	10–15	—	—
Abdominal	0.0625% bupivacaine +2–5 μg/ml fentanyl	4–6	3–4	10–15	—	—
	0.125% bupivacaine + 0.5 μg/ml sufentanil	3–5	2–3	10–15	—	—
	0.1–0.2% ropivacaine + 2–5 μg/ml fentanyl	3–5	2–5	10–15	—	—
	0.125% bupivacaine + 0.05–0.1 mg/ml morphine	4–6	10	15–20	—	—
Lower extremity	0.0625–0.125% bupivacaine +2–5 μg/ml fentanyl	4	2	10–15	—	—

Table 4. PCEA regimen for acute postsurgery pain.

Type of surgery	Catheter location	Continuous infusion rate (ml/h)
Thoracic	T2-T9	4–10
Upper abdominal	T4-L1	4–10
Lower abdominal	T10-L3	8–18
Lower extremity	T12-L3	8–18

Table 5. Common continuous infusion rates for epidural analgesia.

numbness in areas other than the operative site and unpredictable effect due to individual anatomic variation [6–30].

Regional anesthesia can be given as continuous block and demand dose using patient-controlled regional anesthesia (PCRA). Commonly, PCRA is used in brachial plexus block, sciatic nerve block, and femoral nerve block. PCRA can decrease the consumption of local anesthesia without increasing the pain and high satisfaction level of patient who has undergone total hip or knee arthroplasty compared with continuous infusion. This method should be able to reduce motor block, minimize block of sensory, and better control from breakthrough pain [30–32]. The recommendation for PCRA setting is low basal infusion rate with 4–6 ml/h. for lower extremity and 6–10 ml/h. for upper extremity along with 2–10 ml small bolus doses with 20–60 min lockout interval [5, 31–35].

3.2.1. Drug of choice

All local anesthetics can be used, although the common choice is the short-acting drugs such as lidocaine and prilocaine. Tachyphylaxis has been reported and this condition is associated with occasional cyanosis caused by methemoglobinemia. Perhaps, it is for this reason that the drug is less favored. Bupivacaine, levobupivacaine, and ropivacaine have all been used for continuous peripheral nerve block (CPNB), but in general, there is no enough data available to suggest the best local anesthetic. Some experts suggest that ropivacaine is preferred because it has the capacity to maintain motor function. Casati preferred ropivacaine compared to lidocaine for this reason. However, the evidence for this CPNB difference is limited and varied. For example, 0.2% ropivacaine provides the same pain relief rate when used in interscalene CPNB after shoulder surgery when compared with 0.15% bupivacaine or 0.11% levobupivacaine, but greater motor blockade is obtained. Comparison between bupivacaine and levobupivacaine was not found to be a significant difference. Similar studies doubled the concentration of these drugs (0.25% levobupivacaine compared with 0.25 and 0.4% ropivacaine) showing that analgesia and motor block effects for interscalene catheters were similar at 0.25% levobupivacaine and 0.4% ropivacaine, but better than 0.25% ropivacaine. In a popliteal infusion study, Casati et al. also showed that 0.125% levobupivacaine was roughly equivalent to 0.2% of ropivacaine, either from analgesia or motor block sparing effect [33–39].

The term "analgesic gap" has been used for periods of inadequate analgesia that often occur after the loss of the initial block effect associated with catheter placement, but before subsequent local anesthetic infusions produce full effect. It may be especially difficult to treat if the patient is discharged after an outpatient operation with a catheter and infusion system. Keep in mind that regular oral analgesia should be started before the block runs out, and additional analgesia is readily available and used as early as the patient begins to feel uncomfortable with the pain.

Despite the recently published preclinical evidence of perineural pregabalin infusions and addition of clonidine, dexamethasone, and buprenorphine in perineural bupivacaine injected in mice, these data are still premature and until now there has been no drug other than local anesthesia approved by the FDA for continuous perineural administration. Randomized controlled clinical trials have failed to show the advantage of adding clonidine or epinephrine to perineural infusions. There are sporadic RCTs that show the benefits of some opioids in perineural infusions, but all these studies lack the active systemic control group that cannot assess the importance of perineural vs. intravenous opioid drug delivery. On the other hand, the addition of opioids often leads to an increased incidence of opioid-related side-effects. Recent data support previous evidence showing that total doses, not concentration/volume, are a major factor affecting clinical effects for continuous infusion of peripheral nerves [33, 35, 38–40].

3.2.2. PCRA brachial plexus

Insertion of brachial plexus catheter is generally divided into four parts: interscalene, supraclavicular, infraclavicular, and axillary. Choosing the right location for the insertion of the catheter in certain surgical procedures is of great importance compared to considering the variety of anesthesia techniques to be used.

3.2.2.1. PCRA axillary nerve block

After elective surgery on the hands, continuous axillary blocks using 0.1 or 0.2% ropivacaine did not have a better effect when compared to a control group using saline, and both groups still need additional analgesia. However, both in the continuous group and the recurrent bolus dose group using the 0.25% bupivacaine regimen gave better results in relieving pain with no difference in the two groups with the different techniques, either on the pain score, motor block degree, or on opioid requirements, although plasma bupivacaine levels were higher in the continuous group. Both 0.125% bupivacaine and 0.125% ropivacaine, given as a 10-ml patient-controlled bolus dosage in outpatients, can relieve pain equally well. In addition to pain relief, continuous axillary block can provide an increased effect of vascular flow in patients after fingers reimplantation surgery [33, 39, 41].

3.2.2.2. PCRA brachial plexus periclavicular (supraclavicular/infraclavicular)

The periclavicular area has the advantage for the placement of a brachial plexus catheter. Unlike the axilla, this area is cleaner and relatively with less movement. With the increasing popularity of the infraclavicular block, various approaches of plexus catheterization are also increasingly used. The infraclavicular catheter has been widely used to relieve postoperative pain in the arms, elbows, and hands, even in patients undergoing outpatient treatment. Ilfeld et al. compared the use of ropivacaine infusions in the infraclavicular brachial plexus compared with normal saline use in patients undergoing postsurgical upper-limb care treatment; patients receiving ropivacaine infusions experienced fewer pain complaints, fewer sleep disturbances, and used less opioids, resulting in fewer opioid side effects, and higher patient satisfaction [31, 33, 39, 42].

3.2.2.3. PCRA interscalene brachialis

Shoulder surgery can be very painful. Early and effective rehabilitation is important in improving postoperative outcomes. Given the substantial restriction of rehabilitation, it may not be surprising that the subject of local anesthetic infusion through the interscalene catheter is a new discussion in the literature on continuous peripheral nerve blocks and their use for pain relief following major surgery on the shoulders that has been widespread. The growing evidence now confirms that, in general, continuous interscalene brachial plexus may provide superior analgesia than intravenous opioids. For example, patient-controlled interscalene analgesia or continuous infusion of interscalene analgesia may ease pain, increase patient satisfaction, reduce opioid side effects compared with analgesia with IV-PCA and oral opioid analgesia. Interscalene analgesia also eases pain better and reduces opioid need after shoulder surgery compared with single injection interscalene block and infusion of local anesthesia into the glenohumeral joint or subacromial bursa, although mild adverse events may increase. For the record, it is worth mentioning that the most popular skin area for catheter access placement to the interscalene brachial plexus is also relatively mobile. For this reason, some anesthesiologists who use this technique will direct the catheter to the skin that is not moving much using tunneling technique [31, 33–35, 37, 39, 43–45].

3.2.2.4. Regimen dose

Some experts have used a number of different infusion strategies, ranging from simple continuous infusion rates, or controlled by patients, intermittent dose of bolus on demand only, to a combination of the two. The optimal local anesthetic regimen for CPNB is a combination of continuous infusion and patient-controlled bolus dosage which is known as patient controlled regional analgesia (PCRA). Grossi and Allegri and several other studies concluded that the best infusion regimen is a combination of continuous basal infusion with minimal rate, along with an intermittent bolus on demand that would otherwise result in a lower total local anesthetic use, than a continuous infusion course at a rate relatively with high infusion with equally effective analgesia results. There is insufficient evidence for optimal infusion rates, bolus doses on demand, or lockout intervals, although continuous infusion rates of 4–10 ml/h, bolus dose on demand 2–5 ml, and 20–60 min lockout interval have been successfully used. However, there will always be variations between patients, and the regimen should be adjusted to give the desired effect [33, 35, 37, 39, 41–46].

Currently, no known maximum safe dose for long-acting local anesthetics is administered continuously or via PCRA. In some studies, involving patients without kidney or liver disease, perineural infusions for 5 days with scheduled times indicate that the concentration of the drug in the blood is at a safe level. Administration of bupivacaine may be considered at a maximum infusion rate of 0.5 mg/kg/h based on predictions from data of patients receiving epidural bupivacaine infusion. Patients undergoing shoulder surgery using an interscalene catheter, supplemental block with large bolus dose (6 ml) can decrease continuous infusion rate from 8 to 4 ml/h and may prolong the duration of the infusion. However, many incidents and increased intensity of breakthrough pain, sleep disorders, and decreased pain management satisfaction were reported. Therefore, if outpatients do not regain control to obtain additional local anesthesia, practitioners experience a dilemma regarding the use of analgesia selected between strong analgesia for a shorter period of time or weaker analgesia for a longer period of time. For the record, the duration of the infusion may be increased by progressively decreasing the basal infusion rate with a programmable infusion pump, thereby theoretically maximizing postoperative analgesia [33, 35, 37, 39, 41–46].

Different results in doses of drug regimens can be caused by various factors, such as catheter design (no stimulation vs. stimulation), catheter placement (ultrasound vs. stimulation vs. combination) techniques, local anesthetic types (ropivacaine vs. bupivacaine vs. levobupivacaine) and concentration, infusion basal rate, bolus volume, lockout interval, operating procedures, yield evaluation, measurement sensitivity, and many other factors. As a result, there is no evidence-based regimen that is ideal, although researchers have provided clinical recommendations. However, there are some clinical situations where bolus dose administration is theoretically useful such as increasing block strength before wound care or potentially painful physical therapy. An RCT study showed that bolus on demand at PCRA reduced the need for local anesthesia. This provides three possible advantages: (1) theoretically reduces the motor block by decreasing the required basal infusion rate (to date, there is insufficient research), (2) reducing the incidence of numbness in the extremities, and (3) increasing the duration of the infusion/analgesia for outpatients who are dismissed from hospital with predetermined local anesthetic reservoir volume [31, 33, 37, 39, 43, 44, 46].

Some patients, especially the geriatrics, will experience a decrease in postoperative cognitive impairment. Therefore, most practitioners provide education to patients with their family/caregiver. They should be given oral and written instructions, along with contact numbers of health workers who can be contacted. In addition to standard outpatient instructions, the items described include the after effects of anesthesia, instructions on the infusion pump, management of breakthrough pain, care of peripheral nerve catheters, the protection of limbs, and plans for catheter release. In addition, it is necessary to inform the onset of pain in the operative limb after the loss of peripheral nerve block effects, the possibility of fluid leakage at the site of the catheter and its treatment, and possible complications such as nerve injury, local infection, toxicity of local anesthetics, and pulmonary disorders. One variation of the technique that recently attracted attention was the use of mandated/programmed intermittent bolus (PIB) doses, using the theoretical basis that increased local anesthetic volumes administered at one time that could increase perineural spread compared to volume/dose equivalent given as a basal infusion. Continuous adductor channel block requires a higher local basal anesthetic rate than the femoral nerve block. One study showed that although local anesthetic agents were given at relatively high rates (8 ml/h), the spread of local anesthetics remained limited. Subsequent studies involving healthy volunteers showed 0.2% ropivacaine at 8 ml/h as basal dose or intermittent bolus doses hourly gave the same sensory perceptions and quadriceps strength. Similar results are also reported for interscalene, femoral, and popliteal/sciatic catheters. For these reasons, the use of recurrent bolus doses can be reduced, unless recent RCTs may demonstrate the benefit of analgesia after thoracotomy at relatively

Surgery procedure	Anesthesia intraoperative	Postoperative PCRA			
		Medicine	Continuous (ml/h)	Bolus on demand (ml)	Lockout interval (min)
Shoulder surgery	Interscalene catheter: 20–25 ml ropivacaine 0.5% or 15–20 ml bupivacaine 0.5% + epinephrine 1:300,000 or 15–20 ml levobupivacaine 0.5%	Ropivacaine 0.2%	0–5 (child: 0.02 ml/kg)	2–5 (child: 0.1 ml/kg)	15–30
		Bupivacaine 0.1–0.125%	0–6	2–5	20–60
		Levobupivacaine 0.1–0.2%	0–6	2–5	20–60
Upper and lower arm surgery	Infraclavicular or supraclavicular catheter: 20–25 ml ropivacaine 0.5% or 15–20 ml bupivacaine 0.5% + epinephrine 1:300,000 or 15–20 ml levobupivacaine 0.5%	Ropivacaine 0.2%	0–5 (child: 0.02 ml/kg)	2–5 (child: 0.1 ml/kg)	15–30
		Bupivacaine 0.1–0.125%	0–6	2–5	20–60
		Levobupivacaine 0.1–0.2%	0–6	2–5	20–60
Lower arm and hand surgery	Axillary: 15–20 ml bupivacaine 0.5% or 15–20 ml levobupivacaine 0.5%	Bupivacaine 0.25%	0–10	2–10	30–60
		Levobupivacaine 0.1–0.2%	0–10	2–10	30–60

Table 6. List of surgery, operative anesthesia, and postoperative analgesia.

large levobupivacaine (15 ml) volumes via paravertebral catheters, every 6 h compared with continuous infusions [33, 42, 44, 46] (**Table 6**).

3.2.3. *PCRA femoral nerve*

The femoral nerve block is particularly indicated for pain control associated with unilateral anterior knee surgery. It is important to remember that the posterior obturator nerve provides an articular branch that supplies the posterior aspect of the knee, and this nerve may contribute to the pain that occurs in the posterior aspect of the knee after knee surgery, even though the femoral nerve block is effective. Therefore, additional sciatic nerve block is required if surgery is performed in the distal or posterior areas of the knee joint (e.g., on anterior or posterior cruciate ligament repair). It is not uncommon to require obturator nerve blocks and/or sciatic nerve separately, in addition to the femoral nerve block after total knee replacement surgery. Often the pain experienced in the posterior knee is short and effectively controlled with a single injection block. Continuous femoral nerve block has been shown to improve postoperative outcomes of total knee arthroplasty, better than single-shot femoral nerve block and continuous epidural [33, 35–39, 46–49].

For early bolus injections, 0.25 ml/kg ropivacaine (0.25–0.5%) or bupivacaine (0.25–0.5%) as bolus injection for intra- and postoperative analgesia should be combined with general anesthesia. If used as a single anesthetic, a dose of 0.5 ml/kg is usually required. With this technique, breakthrough pain is rare, and patients feel comfortable when followed by a continuous dose of 0.1 ml/kg/h in children or 5 ml/h in adults with 0.25% ropivacaine or bupivacaine 0.25%. The use of PCRA can give a better effect. Increased PCRA requirements are often caused by improper catheter placement [33, 37, 38, 47, 48, 50–52] (**Table 7**).

http://dx.doi.org/10.5772/intechopen.79302

Local anesthesia	PCA setting			PIB	
	Continuous (ml/h)	Bolus (ml)	Lockout (min)	Volume (ml)	Interval (every)
Bupivacaine 0.1–0.25%	0–10 (child: 0.1 ml/kg//h)	5–10	30–60	–	–
Ropivacaine 0.2–0.25%	2–8 (child: 0.1 ml/kg/h)	4–15	30–60	30	4 h
				5–10	60–75 min
Levobupivacaine 0.125–0.25%	**0–5**	5–10	20–30	–	–

Table 7. Setting of PCRA with catheter in femoral nerve.

3.2.4. PCRA sciatic nerve

The sciatica nerve block is particularly indicated for pain management associated with unilateral ankle, and in cases of lower leg operation. It is important to note that the saphenous nerves supply the medial aspect of the lower legs, ankles, and even the soles, which are branches of the femoral nerve. A single injection sciatica nerve block usually lasts relatively long, up to 36 h and continuous nerve blocks may be indicated for special cases. Arthroplasty surgery on the ankle is a good example requiring a sciatica nerve block. If necessary, it can be combined with a saphenous nerve block. For early bolus injections, 0.25 ml/kg of ropivacaine 0.2–0.5% or 0.2–0.5% bupivacaine may be used as bolus injection for intra- and postoperative analgesia if block is combined with general anesthesia. If used as a single anesthetic, a dose of 0.5 ml/kg is usually required. With this technique, breakthrough pain is very rare, and patients feel comfortable when followed by a continuous dose of 0.1 ml/kg/h in children or 5 ml/h in adults with 0.25% ropivacaine or bupivacaine 0.25%. The use of PCRA can give a better effect. High PCRA demands are often caused by improper catheter placement. In continuous popliteal sciatic block, local anesthetic administered as a programmed intermittent bolus (PIB) in conjunction with PCA provided similar pain relief as a continuous infusion technique combined with PCA. However, the new dosing regimen reduced the need for additional PCA and the overall total consumption of local anesthetic [33, 36, 39, 46, 47, 49, 53, 54] (**Table 8**).

The home release of patients with a peripheral nerve catheter can be performed by various techniques such as the patient may be discharged with written instructions, the health worker

Location of sciatic catheter	Local anesthesia	Setting of PCA		
		Continuous (ml/h)	Bolus on demand (ml)	Lockout interval (min)
Subgluteus	Ropivacaine 0.2%	5–10 (child: 0.1 ml/kg/h)	5–10	30–60
Anterior	Ropivacaine 0.2%	5–6	5–10	15–30
Popliteal	Ropivacaine 0.2%	8–12	4–10	30–60
	Levobupivacaine 0.125%	3–10	3–5	15–60

Table 8. PCRA setting with catheter in sciatic nerve (with or without femoral nerve block).

may perform this procedure, or the patient's caregiver (or sometimes the patient himself) can release the catheter with instructions provided by healthcare workers via telephone. Among these techniques, there are no procedures that are superior to others. Based on one of the surveys, 98% of patients feel comfortable removing their own catheters at home by giving instructions via telephone. Only 4% chose to return to health workers to remove catheters, and 43% felt comfortable with written instructions. Nonsterile gloves need to be given to patients if they intend to remove their own catheter at home. However, if the catheter is done by stitching fixation, then it should be removed only by medical personnel [33].

3.3. Field blocks

3.3.1. Transversus abdominis plane block (TAP block)

The TAP block is a novel technique for postoperative analgesia especially in the initial postoperative period. TAP block is a technique of locoregional anesthesia that involves the abdominal wall. This block was recently introduced for operations that involve the abdominal wall. The local anesthetic is placed in the plane between transversus abdominis muscle (TAM) and the internal oblique muscle (IOM), where there are sensorial afferent bundles of the nerves T7 to T12 and L1. The local anesthetic injected in the plane blocks the sensory afferents of all these nerves, providing pain relief for the entire anterior abdominal wall. Postoperative pain is an important issue with abdominoplasty and flank liposuction procedures. Bupivacaine hydrochloride (0.5%, 5 mg/ml, total dose, 2 mg/kg), 0.5% lignocaine, 0.375% bupivacaine 20 ml, levobupivacaine to a maximum dose of 1 mg/kg each side, and 0.75% ropivacaine up to 1.5 mg/kg (to a maximum dose of 150 mg) or other local anesthetics are injected bilaterally in the plane between the internal oblique muscles and the transversus abdominis muscles using a blunt needle, with or without USG guidance or injected directly during the surgical procedure. Doses were increased in order to provide prolonged postoperative analgesia. Prolonged analgesic effect can be achieved by continuous blockade using catheter for drug delivery, but it is technically more demanding. For abdominal plastic surgery, TAP block to control postoperative pain administered after the flap resection and prior to the muscles plication. TAP block is used in esthetic abdominoplasty and postbariatric surgery. Compared between these two surgical procedures, TAP block gives better pain control in esthetic abdominoplasty than in postbariatric surgery. The larger amount of tissue resected in bariatric surgery gives greater stimulation of pain fiber. TAP block technique is associated with low postoperative requirements for morphine or other pain medication. It has got potential to substitute the use of intravenous opioid analgesics and hence to avoid its complications. It has been proved to cater significant analgesic effect especially below T10 up to L1 level [55–59].

The TAP block can be done either in preoperative or in postoperative, but because the abdominal wall is intact preoperatively, it is preferred to be done before the surgery. The procedure must be done under extreme aseptic technique due to the risk of peritoneum penetration. The patient is positioned supine in both techniques [60]. There are two common techniques for TAP block [57–61]: (1) The blind TAP: the point of entry for the blind TAP is the lumber triangle of Petit. The needle is inserted cephalad to the iliac crest and advanced until two distinct "pops" are felt as the needle transverses the external oblique and internal oblique muscles. To make the loss of resistance more appreciable, it is recommended to use a blunt needle.

(2) The ultrasound-guided TAP: the ultrasound probe is placed midway between the costal margin and the iliac crest to image in the transverse plane. The muscle layers are identified on the ultrasound image. The needle is gradually passed through the skin, subcutaneous tissue, EO, and IO, until it lies between the IO and TA—this is where the local anesthetic should be injected (**Figure 4** and **Table 9**).

3.3.2. Continuous wound infusion system

Continuous wound infusion of local anesthetic will block the transmission of nociceptive stimuli from the wound surface, inhibit response of local inflammation to surgical wound, and suppress the spinal cord from systemic absorption of local anesthetics. Currently, this special wound infusion catheter can be inserted intra- and perioperatively into the wound. Liu et al. performed a meta-analysis on the available randomized controlled trials (RCTs). Forty-four prospective randomized trials met the inclusion criteria for analysis. Overall results and

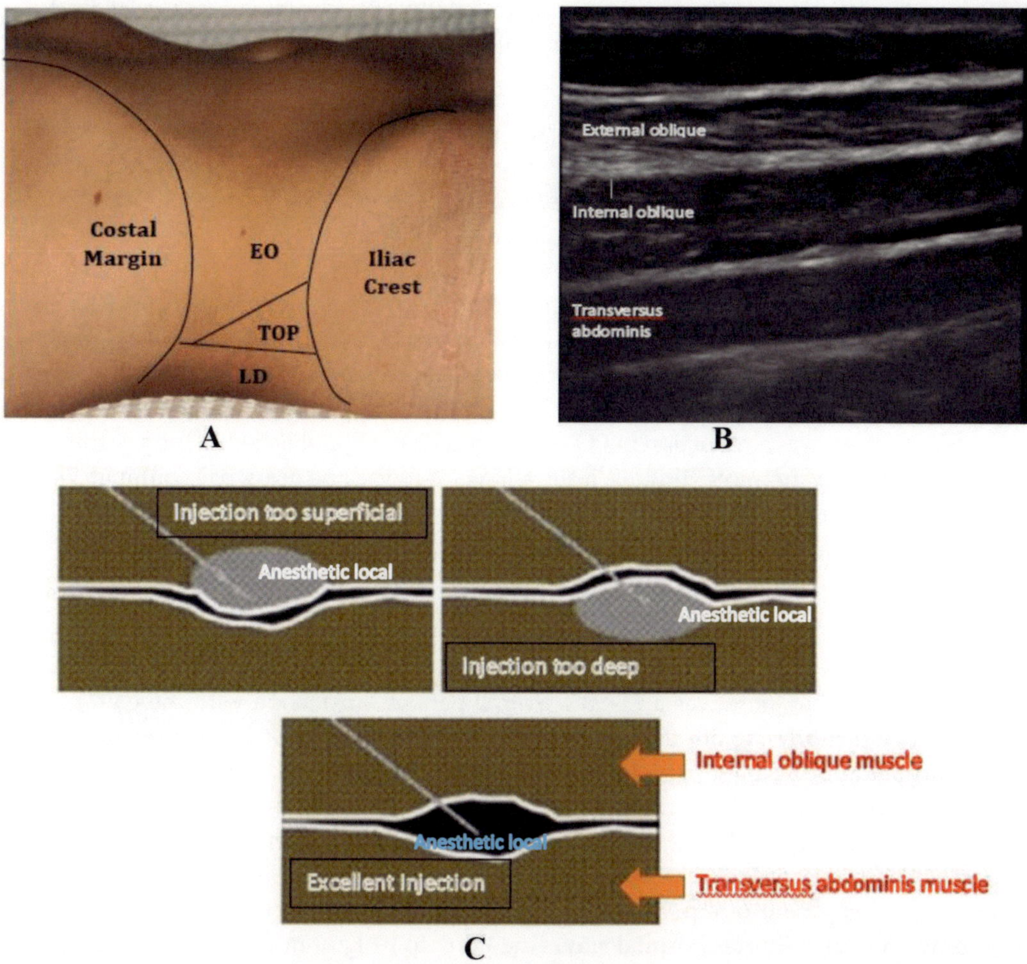

Figure 4. Landmark (a), USG guide (b), and location of TAP injection (c) [60].

Complications	Contraindications	
	Absolute	Relative
Local anesthetic toxicity	Patient refusal	Coagulopathy
Intraperitoneal injection	Allergy to local anesthetic	Surgery at injection site
Bowel injury	Localized infection over injection point	
Hepatic injury		

Table 9. Complication and contraindication of TAP block [60].

all subgroup analysis showed that continuous local anesthetic infusion improved pain scores and decreased the need for supplemental narcotics. These results were statistically significant. Another randomized controlled trials had been done to examine the efficacy of this system in pain management, from the trials when compared with placebo, and this system can reduce the pain score as much as 33%. It is recommended that in the absence of neuraxial blocks or peripheral nerve blocks, wound infiltration should be performed whenever possible [6, 62–65].

To deliver continuous wound infusion, we can use a pain pump that has been studied in various types of surgical procedures. Although pain pumps have been used in many surgical procedures, their use is relatively new in plastic surgery. The catheter is placed in the surgical site and local anesthetics are delivered to the site. Typically, using 0.25% bupivacaine or 0.25–0.5% ropivacaine can be infused continuously, bolused, or delivered via a patient-controlled delivery system. The 0.25% bupivacaine is usually infused at 2 ml/h for 48 h, delivering 120 mg per day. This is well below the recommended maximum dose of 400 mg in 24 h [6, 62, 63, 65, 66]. Baroody et al. [67], in a study of 16 patients with autologous latissimus dorsi breast reconstruction with historical controls, showed that continuous infusion of 0.25% bupivacaine, 2.08 ml/h, decreased pain level and significantly used less opioid in the postoperative period. They also observed that there was a reduction in PONV. Lu and Fine [68] published a study of the use of indwelling catheters for the continuous infiltration of bupivacaine using pain pump in 74 consecutive breast reductions and 74 consecutive tissue expander breast reconstruction patients, and each group was compared with patients receiving conventional analgesia. Pain and average pain score was significantly lower, but do not eliminate pain, in the pain pump group than in the comparison group, as were cumulative amounts of pain medications. There were no statistically significant differences in the number of complications or in the rate of PONV.

One study found that there was a 91–93% overall patient satisfaction with the pain pumps, which was statistically significantly greater than the saline group satisfaction rate. There was significant improvement in patient satisfaction in the bupivacaine group, and their PCA narcotic use was decreased in the first 48 h [62]. Giordano et al. [69] in their study about abdominal donor site analgesia in patients undergoing free lower abdominal flap breast reconstruction comparing pain pump use vs. control found a significantly decreased use of opioids after using pain pump vs. control and a trend toward reduction in the antiemetic medicament use and shorter hospital stay. One thing to be kept in mind is that the surgeon and anesthetist must be aware of the risk of local anesthetic systemic toxicity, although it is very rare. Care must be taken not to exceed the daily maximum dose of local anesthetics, including the amount infiltrated with surgery as well as the total amount infused via the pain pump [62, 66, 70, 71]. Even though pain pump is popular, the cost-effectiveness of these pain pumps needs further investigation.

3.3.3. *Tumescent analgesia*

Tumescent analgesia (TA) is a part of local anesthesia using a very dilute local anesthetic, which delivered subcutaneously in a large volume of fluid. In plastic surgery, TA can be used alone or with sedation to achieve intraoperative analgesia. It can also be used along with neuraxial analgesia or general anesthesia to get postoperative analgesia and lower intraoperative anesthesia. This technique was used most commonly in liposuction, but can also be used in other plastic surgeries such as subcutaneous mass excisions and scar revisions, excisional body contouring (abdominoplasty, body lifts, arm lifts, and thigh lifts), breast augmentation, reduction, mastopexy, gynecomastia, and capsular contracture revision, mastectomy, burn excision and skin grafting, skin procedures (dermabrasion and laser resurfacing), face and neck lifts, and hair grafting. TA can be used in other procedures to decrease intra- and postoperative pain, allowing less use or elimination of anesthesia and opioids. The addition of diluted epinephrine in TA leads to vasoconstriction that can significantly lower the blood loss, minimizing bruising, and postoperative soreness. The advantages of TA are fewer narcotic use, less sedation, and less general anesthesia needed, faster recovery, and earlier discharge. These advantages could prevent the use of general anesthesia and decrease the possibility of pulmonary thromboembolism [72–76].

TA fluid formula is based on 1000 ml of either 0.9% saline or ringer lactate solution. When the tumescent technique is used with general anesthesia, the concentration of epinephrine is 1:1,000,000. This solution can be added with bupivacaine, lidocaine, hyaluronidase, or triamcinolone 10 mg/L and has also been used to decrease ecchymosis and edema, but there is a little comparative evidence regarding its usefulness. Lidocaine is most commonly used as a local anesthetic in TA. The recommended maximum dose of lidocaine used for TA is different compared to a traditional local infiltration (**Table 10**). Bupivacaine can be used alone or with lidocaine. A patient who received bupivacaine has a shorter hospital stay. If the patient is allergic to lidocaine, prilocaine can be used instead. The recommended dose of prilocaine of 8 mg/kg for small volume liposuction and doses up to 35 mg/kg is safe. Patient should be monitored for 12 h after administration of prilocaine to evaluate if there are methemoglobinemia sign and symptoms such as a headache, dyspnea, lightheadedness, weakness, confusion, delirium, palpitations, chest pain, cyanosis, dysrhythmias, seizures, coma, acidosis, and cardiac or neurologic ischemia and should be precautious in liver patients [72–76].

Tumescent fluid is administered with an 18G long spinal needle for a small procedure or blunt infiltration cannula for the larger procedures. Before TA is given, lidocaine 1% and 1:100,000 epinephrine is injected intradermally to decrease skin bleeding. Plasma peak of lidocaine is seen 10–14 h after its administration, but in the highly vascularized area, the peak of lidocaine reaches in 6 h. Monitoring should be extended in a patient who receives high dose of lidocaine. Lidocaine toxicity is suspected in a patient with restlessness, drowsiness, light-headedness, metallic taste, tinnitus, slurred speech, and numbness in lips and tongue, shivering, muscle twitching, tremors followed by convulsion, central nervous system depression, coma, respiratory depression, and cardiac arrest. If signs of toxicity appear, stop infusion of fluids with

Medication	Concentration (%)	Maximum dose range		
		Without epinephrine (mg/kg) for TA	With epinephrine (mg/kg) for TA	"Traditional local infiltration" dose with and without epinephrine (mg/kg)
Lidocaine	1.0	30–60	90–120	4–7
Bupivacaine	0.25	120–240	180	2.5–3
Ropivacaine	0.2	120–360	120–360	2.7
Mepivacaine	1.0	45–90	120	4–7
Etidocaine	0.5	120–180	180	4–5.5
Epinephrine (1:1000)	1:1000	0.5–2 ml of 1:1000		
Sodium bicarbonate (8.4%)	8.4	10–12.5 ml		—

Table 10. Common tumescent analgesia concentration and dose.

local anesthetics, protect airway and oxygenation, call for help, and give benzodiazepines if seizures happened. Manage arrhythmia based on ACLS guidelines but avoid lidocaine, give lipid emulsion therapy if cardiac or neurological event persists [70–73].

Discomfort during injection of lidocaine can be decreased with the addition of sodium bicarbonate. Sodium bicarbonate is contraindicated as addition to bupivacaine because it can precipitate the solution. High volumes of TA infusion have a risk of intravascular fluid overload with cardiac and pulmonary effect. In a patient with cardiac, pulmonary, or renal pathology, the pros and cons of TA must be considered with the limitation of the injected volume. Patient with high-volume TA can have a risk of mild hyponatremia and hypokalemia, lowering body temperature with impaired thermoregulatory system, and acute nerve compression. Administration of TA at 37°C can decrease the risk of hypothermia. In a patient with nerve compression, this condition can be resolved after giving diuretics [72, 73].

4. Conclusion

The patients who undergo plastic surgery procedure can experience various types of pain, including background pain, breakthrough pain, and procedural pain. Treatment for each type of plastic surgery and resulted pain requires a specific approach and must be individualized to the patient. There are three main techniques in acute pain management postoperatively, such as systemic analgesia, regional analgesia, and local/topical analgesia. Currently, pain management through intravenous injection or continuous central neuraxial and peripheral nerve block is more controllable and safer since the invention of pain pump, which commonly use the principal of patient-controlled analgesia. Multimodal treatment seems to have significant benefits, postoperative dosing becomes more complex, and adverse drug interactions and drug overdose become more likely. There is some combination that has demonstrated a good effect in multimodal analgesia. PCA intravenous, patient-controlled epidural analgesia (PCEA) and patient-controlled regional analgesia (PCRA) can be combined with other pain killers, such as paracetamol, NSAIDs, alpha-2-delta modulators (gabapentin and pregabalin), N-methyl-D-aspartate (NMDA) antagonists (ketamine and magnesium), alpha-2-agonists (clonidine and dexmedetomidine), TAP block, continuous wound infusion system using pain pump, and tumescent analgesia with local anesthetic.

Author details

I Gusti Ngurah Mahaalit Aribawa*, Made Wiryana, Tjokorda Gde Agung Senapathi and Pontisomaya Parami

*Address all correspondence to: mahaalit@unud.ac.id

Department of Anesthesiology and Intensive Care, Udayana University, Badung, Indonesia

References

[1] Aribawa IGNM, Wiryana M, Parami P, Senapathi TGA. Pain Management in Plastic Surgery. London: IntechOpen; 2018. DOI: 10.5772/intechopen.79302

[2] Banicek J, Acute BD. Acute pain management following roux-en-Y gastric bypass. Surgery. 2011;**25**(18):59-65. DOI: 10.7748/ns2011.01.25.18.35.c8232

[3] Benzon HT, Ratmell JP, Wu CL, Turk DC, Argoff CE, Hurley RW. Practical Management of Pain. 5th ed. Philadelphia: Elsevier Inc; 2014

[4] Faucher L, Furukawa K. Practice guidelines for the management of pain. Journal of Burn Care and Research. 2006;**27**(5):659-668

[5] Macintyre PE, Schug SA. Acute Pain Management: A Practical Guide. 4th ed. Boca Raton, Florida: CRC Press; 2015

[6] Joshi GP. Putting it all together: Recommendations for improving pain management in plastic surgical procedures. Plastic and Reconstructive Surgery. 2014;**134**:94S-100S. DOI: 10.1097/PRS.0000000000000677

[7] Chou R, Gordon DB, De Leon-Casasola OA, Rosenberg JM, Bickler S, Brennan T, et al. Management of postoperative pain: A clinical practice guideline from the American pain society, the American society of regional anesthesia and pain medicine, and the American society of anesthesiologists' committee on regional anesthesia, executive commi. The Journal of Pain. 2016;**17**(2):131-157. DOI: 10.1016/j.jpain.2015.12.008

[8] Elvir-Lazo OL, White PF. Postoperative pain management after ambulatory surgery: Role of multimodal analgesia. Anesthesiology Clinics. 2010;**28**(2):217-224. DOI: 10.1016/j.anclin.2010.02.011

[9] Apfelbaum JL, Ashburn MA, Gan TJ, Nickinovich DG. Practice guidelines for acute pain management in the perioperative setting. An updated report by the American Society of Anesthesiologists Task Force on acute pain management. Anesthesiology. 2012;**116**(2):248-273. DOI: 10.1097/ALN.0b013e31823c1030

[10] Gan TJ, Meyer T, Apfel CC, Chung F, Davis PJ, Eubanks S, et al. Consensus guidelines for managing postoperative nausea and vomiting. Anesthesia and Analgesia. 2003; **97**(1):62-71

[11] Choi BM. A new therapeutic option for postoperative pain management with oxycodone HCI injection. Korean Journal of Anesthesiology. 2016;**69**(3):211-218. DOI: 10.4097/kjae.2016.69.3.211

[12] Kokki H, Kokki M, Sjövall S. Oxycodone for the treatment of postoperative pain. Expert Opinion on Pharmacotherapy. 2012;**13**(7):1045-1058. DOI: 10.1517/14656566.2012.677823

[13] Park J-H, Lee C, Shin Y, An J-H, Ban J-S, Lee J-H. Comparison of oxycodone and fentanyl for postoperative patient-controlled analgesia after laparoscopic gynecological surgery. Korean Journal of Anesthesiology. 2015;**68**(2):153-158. DOI: 10.4097/kjae.2015.68.2.153

[14] Cheung CW, Ying CLA, Lee LHY, Tsang SF, Tsui SL, Irwin MG. An audit of postoperative intravenous patient-controlled analgesia with morphine: Evolution over the last decade. European Journal of Pain. 2009;**13**(5):464-471. DOI: 10.1016/j.ejpain.2008.05.013

[15] Kissin I. Patient-controlled-analgesia analgesimetry and its problems. Anesthesia and Analgesia. 2009;**108**(6):1945-1949. DOI: 10.1213/ane.0b013e3181a1a481

[16] Coniam S, Mendham J. Management of acute pain: Principles and practice - patient controlled analgesia. In: Principles of Pain Management for Anaesthetists. Oxford: Hodder Arnold; 2006. pp. 89-90

[17] Grass JA. Patient-controlled analgesia. Anesthesia and Analgesia. 2005;**101**:44-61

[18] Macintyre PE. Safety and efficacy of patient-controlled analgesia. British Journal of Anaesthesia. 2001;**87**(1):36-46

[19] Pratt N, Tilley P, Schultz D, Lewis S, Vanderveen T, Dharkar-Surber S, et al. San Diego patient safety taskforce tool kit patient controlled analgesia (PCA) guidelines of care. The Journal of the American Medical Association;**2014**:1-16

[20] McNicol E, Ferguson M, Hudcova J. Patient controlled opioid analgesia versus conventional opioid analgesia for postoperative pain. Cochrane Database System Reviews. 2015;**18**(6):CD003348

[21] van der Vyver M, Halpern S, Joseph G. Patient-controlled epidural analgesia versus continuous infusion for labour analgesia: A meta-analysis. British Journal of Anaesthesia. 2002;**89**(3):459-465

[22] Wong CA, Ratliff JT, Sullivan JT, Scavone BM, Toledo P, McCarthy RJ. A randomized comparison of programmed intermittent epidural bolus with continuous epidural infusion for labor analgesia. Anesthesia and Analgesia. 2006;**102**(3):904-909

[23] Capogna G, Camorcia M, Stirparo S, Farcomeni A. Programmed intermittent epidural bolus versus continuous epidural infusion for labor analgesia: The effects on maternal motor function and labor outcome. A randomized double-blind study in nulliparous women. Anesthesia and Analgesia. 2011;**113**(4):826-831. DOI: 10.1213/ANE.0b013e31822827b8

[24] George RB, Allen TK, Habib AS. Intermittent epidural bolus compared with continuous epidural infusions for labor analgesia. Anesthesia and Analgesia. 2013;**116**(1):133-144. DOI: 10.1213/ANE.0b013e3182713b26

[25] Lin Y-N, Zeng F, Li Q, Yang R-M, Liu J-C. The value of programmed intermittent epidural bolus in labor analgesia. Journal of Anesthesia and Critical Care. 2015;**2**(6):1-5

[26] Wu CL, Cohen SR, Richman JM, Rowlingson AJ, Courpas GE, Cheung K, et al. Efficacy of postoperative patient-controlled and continuous infusion epidural analgesia versus intravenous patient-controlled analgesia with opioids: A meta-analysis. Anesthesiology. 2005;**103**(5):1010-1079

[27] Parikh T, Dalwadi D, Divecha V. Comparative study between epidural morphine and bupivacaine with epidural clonidine and bupivacaine for postoperative pain relief in abdominal surgeries. Anesthesia, Essays and Researches. 2015;**9**(1):28-33. DOI: 10.4103/0259-1162.150159

[28] Cook TM, Counsell D, Wildsmith JA. Major complications of central neuraxial block: Report on the third National Audit Project of the Royal College of Anaesthetists. British Journal of Anaesthesia. 2009;**102**(2):179-190. DOI: 10.1093/bja/aen360

[29] Apfelbaum JL. Practice advisory for the prevention, diagnosis, and management of infectious complications associated with neuraxial techniques. Anesthesiology. 2017; **126**(4):585-601. DOI: 10.1097/ALN.0000000000001521

[30] Mannion S, Capdevila X. Peripheral nerve blockade for ambulatory surgery. In: Harmon D, Barret J, Loughnane F, Finucane B, Shorten G, editors. Peripheral Nerve Blocks and Peri-Operative Pain Relief. 2nd ed. Cambridge, UK: Elsevier Inc.; 2010. pp. 60-71

[31] Rawal N, Allvin R, Axelsson K, Hallén J, Ekbäck G, Ohlsson T, et al. Patient-controlled regional analgesia (PCRA) at home: Controlled comparison between bupivacaine and ropivacaine brachial plexus analgesia. Anesthesiology. 2002;**96**(6):1290-1296

[32] Duflo F, Qamouss Y, Rémond C, Pouyau A, Heilporn A, Taylor P, et al. Patient-controlled regional analgesia is effective in children: A preliminary report. Canadian Journal of Anesthesia. 2004;**51**(9):928-930

[33] Ilfeld BM. Continuous peripheral nerve blocks. Anesthesia and Analgesia. 2017;**124**(1): 308-335. DOI: 10.1213/ANE.0000000000001581

[34] Swenson JD, Cheng GS, Axelrod DA, Davis JJ. Ambulatory anesthesia and regional catheters: When and how. Anesthesiology Clinics. 2010;**28**(2):267-280. DOI: 10.1016/j.anclin.2010.02.010

[35] Ilfeld BM. Continuous peripheral nerve blocks in the hospital and at home. Anesthesiology Clinics. 2011;**29**(2):193-211. DOI: 10.1016/j.anclin.2011.04.003

[36] Casati A, Fanelli G, Borghi B, Torri G. Ropivacaine or 2% mepivacaine for lower limb peripheral nerve blocks. Study group on orthopedic anesthesia of the Italian Society of Anesthesia, analgesia, and intensive care. Anesthesiology. 1999;**90**(4):1047-1052

[37] Hanna M, Sloan P. A comparison of levobupivacaine and ropivacaine for interscalene and femoral nerve blocks: A randomized, double-blind, prospective clinical trial. Journal of Anesthesia and Clinical Research. 2011;**2**:5. DOI: 10.4172/2155-6148.1000135

[38] Heid F, Müller N, Piepho T, Bäres M, Giesa M, Drees P, et al. Postoperative analgesic efficacy of peripheral levobupivacaine and ropivacaine: A prospective, randomized double-blind trial in patients after total knee arthroplasty. Anesthesia and Analgesia. 2008;**106**(5):1559-1561. DOI: 10.1213/ane.0b013e318168b493

[39] Chelly JE, Ghisi D, Fanelli A. Continuous peripheral nerve blocks in acute pain management. British Journal of Anaesthesia. 2010;**105**:i86-i96. DOI: 10.1093/bja/aeq322

[40] Jeng CL, Torrillo TM, Rosenblatt MA. Complications of peripheral nerve blocks. British Journal of Anaesthesia. 2010;**105**(Supplement 1):i97-i107. DOI: 10.1093/bja/aeq273

[41] Salonen MH, Haasio J, Bachmann M, Xu M, Rosenberg PH. Evaluation of efficacy and plasma concentrations of ropivacaine in continuous axillary brachial plexus block: High dose for surgical anesthesia and low dose for postoperative analgesia. Regional Anesthesia and Pain Medicine. 2000;**25**(1):47-51

[42] Park SK, Lee SY, Kim WH, Park HS, Lim YJ, Bahk JH. Comparison of supraclavicular and infraclavicular brachial plexus block. Anesthesia and Analgesia. 2017;**124**(2):636-644. DOI: 10.1213/ANE.0000000000001713

[43] Eroglu A. Patient-controlled analgesia after shoulder surgery. Journal of Anesthesia and Critical Care: Open Access. 2014;**1**(3):3-4. DOI: 10.15406/jaccoa.2014.01.00013

[44] Fredrickson MJ, Abeysekera A, Price DJ, Wong AC. Patient-initiated mandatory boluses for ambulatory continuous interscalene analgesia: An effective strategy for optimizing analgesia and minimizing side-effects. British Journal of Anaesthesia. 2011;**106**(2):239-245. DOI: 10.1093/bja/aeq320

[45] Bowens C, Sripada R. Regional blockade of the shoulder: Approaches and outcomes. Anesthesiology Research and Practice. 2012;**2012**:1-12. DOI: 10.1155/2012/971963

[46] Grossi P, Allegri M. Continuous peripheral nerve blocks: State of the art. Current Opinion in Anaesthesiology. 2005;**18**(5):522-526

[47] Anastase DM, Cionac Florescu S, Munteanu AM, Ursu T, Stoica CI. Analgesic techniques in hip and knee arthroplasty: From the daily practice to evidence-based medicine. Anesthesiology Research and Practice. 2014;**2014**:569319. DOI: 10.1155/2014/569319

[48] Boezaart AP. Continuous femoral nerve block. Journal of the New York School of Regional. 2006;**11**:41-47

[49] Boezaart AP. Continuous sciatic nerve block. Journal of the New York School of Regional. 2006;**11**:48-54

[50] Hamp DB, Rod E, Radi A, Granec D, Raki M. Femoral nerve block- or intravenous-guided patient control analgesia for early physical rehabilitation after anterior cruciate ligament reconstruction in "fast-track" orthopedics: What is optimal? Periodicum Biologorum. 2013;**115**(2):219-224

[51] Subramaniam R, Ortho M, Sathappan SS, Ortho F. The effects of single shot versus continuous femoral nerve block on postoperative pain and rehabilitation following total knee arthroplasty. Malaysian Orthopaedic Journal. 2010;**4**(1):19-25

[52] Fowler SJ, Symons J, Sabato S, Myles PS. Epidural analgesia compared with peripheral nerve blockade after major knee surgery: A systematic review and meta-analysis of randomized trials. British Journal of Anaesthesia. 2008;**100**(2):154-164. DOI: 10.1093/bja/aem373

[53] Ilfeld BM, Morey TE, Wang RD, Enneking FK. Continuous popliteal sciatic nerve block for postoperative pain control at home: A randomized, double-blinded, placebo-controlled study. Anesthesiology. 2002;**97**(4):959-965

[54] Taboada M, Rodríguez J, Bermudez M, Amor M, Ulloa B, Aneiros F, et al. Comparison of continuous infusion versus automated bolus for postoperative patient-controlled analgesia with popliteal sciatic nerve catheters. Anesthesiology. 2009;**110**(1):150-154. DOI: 10.1097/ALN.0b013e318191693a

[55] Araco A, Pooney J, Araco F, Gravante G. Transversus abdominis plane block reduces the analgesic requirements after abdominoplasty with flank liposuction. Annals of Plastic Surgery. 2010;**65**(4):385-388. DOI: 10.1097/SAP.0b013e3181cc2a24

[56] Gravante G, Castrì F, Araco F, Araco A. A comparative study of the transversus abdominis plane (TAP) block efficacy on post-bariatric vs aesthetic abdominoplasty with flank liposuction. Obesity Surgery. 2011;**21**(3):278-282. DOI: 10.1007/s11695-010-0203-2

[57] Sforza M, Andjelkov K, Zaccheddu R, Nagi H, Colic M. Transversus abdominis plane block anesthesia in abdominoplasties. Plastic and Reconstructive Surgery. 2011;**128**(2):529-535. DOI: 10.1097/PRS.0b013e31821e6f51

[58] Jankovic Z. Transversus abdominis plane block: The holy grail of anaesthesia for lower abdominal surgery. Periodicum Biologorum. 2009;**111**(2):203-208

[59] Mishra M, Mishra SP. Transversus abdominis plane block: The new horizon for postoperative analgesia following abdominal surgery. Egyptian Journal of Anaesthesia. 2016;**32**:243-247. DOI: doi.org/10.1016/j.egja.2015.12.003

[60] Vlasceanu LG, Constantinescu S, Valcea S, Paduraru DN, Vartic M, Beuran M. TAP block: A new trend in postoperative analgesia after major abdominal surgery? Journal Proceedings of the Romanian Academy Series B. 2015;**S1**:254-257

[61] McDonnell J, ODonnell B, Farrell T, Gough N, Tuite D, Power C, et al. Transversus abdominis plane block: A cadaveric and radiological evaluation. Regional Anesthesia and Pain Medicine. 2007;**32**(5):399-404. DOI: 10.1016/j.rapm.2007.03.011

[62] Chandran GJ, Lalonde DH. A review of pain pumps in plastic surgery. The Canadian Journal of Plastic Surgery. 2010;**18**(1):15-18

[63] Liu SS, Richman JM, Thirlby RC, Wu CL. Efficacy of continuous wound catheters delivering local anesthetic for postoperative analgesia: A quantitative and qualitative

systematic review of randomized controlled trials. Journal of the American College of Surgeons. 2006;**203**(6):914-932. DOI: 10.1016/j.jamcollsurg.2006.08.007

[64] Pu LLQ. Plastic surgery educational foundation DATA committee. The use of a pain pump for optimal postoperative pain management. Plastic and Reconstructive Surgery. 2006;**117**(6):2066-2069. DOI: 10.1097/01.prs.0000210677.44052.3f

[65] Forastiere E, Sofra M, Giannarelli D, Fabrizi L, Simone G. Effectiveness of continuous wound infusion of 0.5% ropivacaine by on-Q pain relief system for postoperative pain management after open nephrectomy. British Journal of Anaesthesia. 2008;**101**(6):841-847. DOI: 10.1093/bja/aen309

[66] Vintar N, Pdbiad C. Wound catheter techniques for postoperative analgesia. Periodicum Biologorum. 2009;**111**(2):227-230

[67] Baroody M, Tameo MN, Dabb RW. Efficacy of the pain pump catheter in immediate autologous breast reconstruction. Plastic and Reconstructive Surgery. 2004;**114**(4). DOI: 895-8-900. doi:10.1097/01.PRS.0000133173.71201.3C

[68] Lu L, Fine NA. The efficacy of continuous local anesthetic infiltration in breast surgery: Reduction mammaplasty and reconstruction. Plastic and Reconstructive Surgery. 2005; **115**(7):1927-34-6

[69] Giordano S, Veräjänkorva E, Koskivuo I, Suominen E. Effectiveness of local anaesthetic pain catheters for abdominal donor site analgesia in patients undergoing free lower abdominal flap breast reconstruction: A meta-analysis of comparative studies. Journal of Plastic Surgery and Hand Surgery. 2013:1-6. DOI: 10.3109/2000656X.2013.788508

[70] Neal JM, Bernards CM, Butterworth JF, Di Gregorio G, Drasner K, Hejtmanek MR, et al. ASRA practice advisory on local anesthetic systemic toxicity. Regional Anesthesia and Pain Medicine. 2010;**35**(2):152-161. DOI: 10.1097/AAP.0b013e3181d22fcd

[71] Dare-Wicker J, Rosenblatt M. Local anesthetic systemic toxicity. In: Anderson MR, Wilson SH, Rosenblatt MA, editors. Decision-Making in Orthopedic and Regional Anesthesiology: A Case-Based Approach. 1st ed. 2015

[72] Gutowski KA. Tumescent analgesia in plastic surgery. Plastic and Reconstructive Surgery. 2014;**134**(4S-2):50S-57S. DOI: 10.1097/PRS.0000000000000678

[73] Klein JA. The tumescent technique for liposuction surgery. American Journal of Cosmetic Surgery. 1987;**4**(4):263-267

[74] Novoa JC. Tumescent anesthetic breast surgery (TABS) [Internet]. Novoa Med Spa. 2011. Available from: http://firstchoicemedicine.com/PerfectImage/pdfs/TABS.pdf

[75] Bennett GD. Anesthesia for liposuction. In: Shiffman MA, Di Giuseppe A, editors. Liposuction: Principles and Practice. 2nd ed. Berlin: Springer; 2016. p. 3-49

[76] Sood J, Jayaraman L, Sethi N. Liposuction: Anaesthesia challenges. Indian Journal of Anaesthesia. 2011;**55**(3):220-227. DOI: 10.4103/0019-5049.82652

Chapter 7

Perioperative Complications in Plastic Surgery

Víctor M. Whizar-Lugo, Jaime Campos-León and Alejandro Moreno-Guillen

Additional information is available at the end of the chapter

http://dx.doi.org/10.5772/intechopen.82269

Abstract

Anesthetic complications in the perioperative period in plastic surgery are extremely rare, although they can be catastrophic and sometimes fatal. The proper selection and correct preoperative assessment of patients are the key to stay away from unwanted events. Preanesthesia evaluation is mandatory in each patient and must include clinical history, complete physical examination, and routine and special laboratory tests in patients with associated pathologies. Anesthetic management is based on these results, type of surgery, experience of the anesthesiologist, and the operating environment. The anesthetic technique can be local, regional, or general with standard noninvasive monitoring. It is recommended that an anesthesiologist be present in all plastic surgery procedures. Complications are usually the result of moving away from the guidelines already established for an excellent practice or the result of sentinel events rather than human errors. Pulmonary embolism is probably the most feared complication, with soft tissue infections being the most frequent complication in plastic surgery. Less common complications include arrhythmias, overhydration, allergies, bleeding, skin necrosis, dehiscence of wounds, brain damage, and dead. Anesthesiologists, surgeons, nurses, and all personnel involved in the care of these patients must work as a team of highly qualified and updated professionals.

Keywords: anesthesia, plastic surgery, perioperative complications

1. Introduction

Patients who consult a plastic surgeon do so with the purpose of improving their body appearance to achieve the image of a beautiful body, increase their self-esteem, and to be more competitive in a globalized world where appearance is a determinant of success. Most are people looking for various alternatives during long time; they search on the Internet, with friends, with patients, in local or distant locations from their place of residence, inside or outside of their country. Some of them make face-to-face consultations with several plastic surgeons before deciding where to have surgery [1]. They seek perfection and full satisfaction to their demands, the best prices, and high expectations with each planned surgical procedure. Complications—small or catastrophic—have no place in the final results. Medical care for these people with special expectancies is a continuous defy, a constant challenge that keeps us at the top of our professional practice and able to achieve excellent results while keeping us competitive in a growing medical market [2, 3]. Fortunately, complications in this clinical environment are rare but often are catastrophic and, to a lesser extent, can be fatal. As in other areas of surgery-anesthesia, adherence to existing guidelines and recommendations is mandatory to avoid any possible unwanted effects.

In recent years, there has been an increase in litigation against the medical profession—justified or not—increasing the costs of health care [4, 5].

The aim of this chapter is to review several aspects related to complications that may occur in the perioperative period of people who undergo plastic surgery procedures under anesthesia.

2. Significant general subjects

In this clinical setting, there are certain general features of paramount importance that should always receive proper attention to avoid unexpected complications. Like any other types of surgical patients, people who desire plastic surgery should be meticulously evaluated regardless of the opinion of the plastic surgeon or the anesthesiologist involved. Standards and guidelines have been described with loose criteria or very strict principles according to the experiences of their authors. The main idea is to study these patients regarding factors that may be important to prevent unfortunate outcomes and staying away from unorthodox practices of our profession [6].

2.1. Optimal preoperative evaluation

The preanesthetic-preoperative assessment is vital and of paramount importance in all patients who undergo plastic surgery. This clinical assessment is an easy, inexpensive, and essential way to decrease catastrophic incidents and complications. Unfortunately, these patients are often considered healthy by their doctors and are not adequately reviewed as determined by the respective certified standards.

During the preanesthetic evaluation, two major groups will be considered; the healthy people and the patients with systemic pathologies that modify their physical conditions (ASA). The evolution and marketing of plastic surgery have generated a third special group of patients—healthy or sick—who travel long distances in search of various aesthetic or reconstructive procedures. This group of patient-tourists has special characteristics that are challenging for the medical group, peculiarities that must be properly evaluated before the patients begin their trip to the surgical destination chosen by them or immediately after their arrival.

Preoperative assessment includes a complete medical history with physical examination. Laboratory and other exams are tailored to each patient depending on their past medical history and findings on previous exams. The current trend is to minimize this type of tests; however, when a perioperative complication occurs and the so-called routine tests (CBC, blood chemistry, blood clotting, blood group) were not carried out, the plaintiffs will have arguments against the medical-surgical team, which is why it is prudent to perform routine exams, leaving the electrocardiogram for hypertensive patients, patients with history of heart disease, diabetics, and healthy people over 50 years old. **Table 1** lists the usual exams for all types of patients.

2.2. Informed consent

The patient, his/her relatives, or companions must be properly informed about the technical aspects and risks of surgery and anesthesia. This document is an indicator of communication between patients and their physicians and should be as complete as possible. While it is almost absurd to mention every risk inherent in each procedure, it is vital to mention the most frequent complications and talk about the possibility of catastrophic mishaps, always leaving

Parameters	ASA 1	ASA 2–3	Observations
Clinical history	Yes	Yes	The general and oriented clinical review made by the anesthesiologist anticipates problems such as difficult airway, spinal anomalies, mental alterations, family environment, and possibility of a lawsuit
Physical examination	Yes	Yes	
Specialist consultation	NE	Yes	It is prudent to know the opinion of the geriatrician, pulmonologist, cardiologist, endocrinologist, surgeon, family therapist in search of polypharmacy, drug interactions, etc.
Electrocardiogram	Only >50 years old	Yes	Arrhythmias, ischemia, growth, or dilatation of heart cavities
Chest X-ray	NE	Yes	Useful in smokers, suspected tuberculosis, neoplasms, emphysema, and kyphosis
Echocardiogram	No	R	Compulsory study in patients with severe arterial hypertension, ischemic patients, and patients with dilated cardiomyopathy
Spirometry	No	R	Its usefulness has not been demonstrated; however, it is recommended in chronic pneumopathy and smokers
Blood test	Yes	Yes	Diagnosis of subclinical anemia
Coagulation tests	Yes	Yes	TP, TPT, INR, and bleeding time are mandatory in anticoagulants, hepatocellular damage, severe sepsis, prolonged fasting, and extreme malnutrition
Complete blood chemistry	Yes	Yes	Kidney, hepatocellular, metabolic and electrolyte evaluation
Urinalysis	NE	Yes	Loss of blood and proteins, changes in urine density
HIV, hepatitis, drugs, and pregnancy	R	R	They are requested based on the clinical history and experience data. HIV is prudent for the protection of medical and paramedical personnel

NE = not essential; R = recommendable.

Table 1. Complete parameters in the preoperative assessment in plastic surgery.

open communication for any questions they might have. Although a well-informed consent does not exempt us from the responsibility of a serious failure, its absence has been a reason of demand in plastic surgery up to 43.8% [5].

2.3. The surgical unit

Surgical units located outside hospitals for outpatient and short-stay procedures in plastic surgery started in the 1960s [7] and rapidly expanded. Currently, most plastic surgeons want to have their own surgical unit. In these surgical units, surgical and nonsurgical procedures are performed; from Botox injection, fillers, CO_2 laser, minimally invasive surgeries such as hair transplantation to major surgeries such as abdominoplasty, breast reconstruction, body contouring procedures in post bariatric patients, and many more. Safety of each patient is the gold standard [8].

Although this type of surgery/anesthesia is valid from a point of view of functionality, resulting in lower costs and generating a higher income, it is prudent to mention that not these surgical units meet the normative requirements, transforming into surgical taverns [7], which could increase the possibility of considerable risks. Performing anesthesia outside a traditional hospital surgical room has gained popularity, and high-risk surgeries on ASA 2 and even some ASA 3 patients are frequently intervened in this area. Sometimes these scenarios are comparable to performing anesthesia outside the operating room [9–11], it is normative to have well-equipped anesthesia machines, standard monitoring (noninvasive blood pressure, electrocardiogram, oximetry, capnography, temperature), monitored recovery area, and well-trained nursing personnel, which ensures a morbidity-mortality rate comparable to that expected in a hospital operating room [10]. It is advisable to have equipment to avoid perioperative hypothermia as well as noninvasive ventilatory assistance equipment. Implementing WHO recommendations in relation to a surgical safety checklist allowed Rosenberg et al. [12] to reduce complications from 11.9 to 2.72% ($p = 0.0006$). These investigators optimized medical resource from 90.9 to 99.5% ($p < 0.0001$). Verbal confirmation on precautions on toxicity by local anesthetics increased from 0 to 91.3% ($p < 0.0001$), among other improvements. These authors also evaluated patient satisfaction, which increased from 57 to 90.8% ($p < 0.0001$). The current surgical room team must balance the safety and comfort of the patient and the medical group; light, sound, climate, air, temperature, humidity, ventilation, drafts, and noise are having a safer, efficient, and more professional environment [13].

The staff of ambulatory surgical units must receive continuing education to keep their certification up-to-date: surgeons, anesthesiologists, nurses, secretaries, and well-qualified administrators are required to ensure excellence. Simulation and educational programs enhance safety and make medical-surgical care systems more effective. Shapiro and his group [14] used a high-fidelity simulator mimicking various critical scenarios in a plastic surgery setting with a special regard to equipment training, communication, crisis, adherence to evidence-based protocols, and regulatory standards. They observed a high degree of acceptance and validity, arousing the participant's interest in the importance of changing processes that improve patient safety and avoid errors. A prospective study on the safety of office-based surgery in Florida and Alabama, USA [15]—where reporting adverse events is mandatory—reviewed complicated events for 10 and 6 years, respectively, and found 46 deaths in Florida and 263 complicated procedures that required moving patients to nearby hospitals;

56.5% (26/46) were deaths and 49.8% (131/263) of the hospital transfers were related to cosmetic surgery. Of these, 67% of deaths and 74% of hospital transfers had been managed under general anesthesia. Liposuction, abdominoplasty with liposuction, and other cosmetic surgeries were related to 10 deaths and 34 hospital transfers. Only 38% of the units reporting adverse events were accredited, 93% of physicians were certified, and 98% had privileges in hospitals. Plastic surgeons reported the most events (45%). In 6 years, in Alabama, there were three deaths and 49 complications and hospital transfers; 42% (22/55) of the transfers and no deaths were associated with cosmetic surgery; 86% were done under general anesthesia. There were only two patients with complicated liposuction who were transferred to the hospital. Unlike units in Florida, 71% of units in Alabama were certified, with 100% certified surgeons. Plastic surgeons reported most events (42.3%). In both states, the complications of dermatologists were minimal or absent because their procedures are less invasive and with local or regional anesthesia. It is desirable that medical groups and health authorities establish a mandatory system that monitors deleterious events in this type of surgical environment to improve current guidelines based on the reality of each country or geographic region studied and can determine the permissible frequency of complicated events in plastic surgery [16].

There are several Government health agencies in charge of the certification of these surgical units that have the common goal of providing a similar and safe environment in this type of establishments. In Mexico, COFEPRIS and the Federal Sanitary System are responsible for verifying the functionality of this type of surgical units; from 2013 to February 2015, verified 1209 clinics provide cosmetic surgery services and found irregularities in 115, and 66 clinics were closed [17]. In the United States of America, the Joint Commission for Accreditation of Hospital Organizations (JCAHO), American Association for Accreditation of Ambulatory Surgery Facility (AAAASF), and American Osteopathic Association's Healthcare Facilities Accreditation Program (HFAP) [18] are the organizations that regulate these aspects.

2.4. Patient safety

Perioperative safety is the primary goal in the comprehensive care of all patients; anesthesiologists, surgeons, nurses, paramedical staff, and health system administrators have developed guidelines aimed at improving safety in this surgical environment by strengthening preventive measures, assessment, pre-trans, and postoperative care to avoid complications. Some groups go beyond the usual recovery time, using pharmacological programs to reduce the incidence of chronic postoperative pain.

In the operating room, patient safety is a shared responsibility between professionals and staff who interact directly or indirectly with patients. As anesthesiologists, our responsibility ranges from patient assessment, anesthesia technique, and immediate recovery, although it can be extended beyond this moment when we use drugs with prolonged pharmacological effects, either as a delayed action or as chronic damage as is the case of arachnoiditis, chronic postoperative pain and perhaps CNS effects of general anesthesia for neonates could be included. Adequate monitoring (cardiorespiratory, temperature, neurological, metabolic, or neuromuscular blocking effects), the position of the patient in the operating table to avoid neurovascular compression injuries, the placement of antiembolic devices, maintenance of normothermia, facial and ocular protection, positioning the head, and avoiding burns and fires are just some of the aspects of which we are responsible during the trans and postoperative period [19–21]. Proper management of the airway is a challenge since there is always the possibility of anatomical anomalies in a patient, which makes it difficult and even impossible to secure an airway.

WHO began its safe surgery program, where checklists have proven their importance in reducing errors. No matter the surgical procedure—small or large—these recommendations list 10 essential objectives: (1) correct surgery site, (2) safe anesthesia, (3) airway management, (4) bleeding management, (5) avoid known allergies, (6) minimize risk of operative infections, (7) prevent the retention of foreign bodies, (8) correct identification of biopsies, (9) effective communication between the surgical team, and (10) systematic surveillance of surgical results. It is advisable to stick to this simple and very effective list. Its implementation is not easy, and it is necessary to understand the nature of the errors, the dynamics that exist between the systems and the people, as well as to create a culture that stimulates the patient's safety [22–24]. In plastic surgery, it should be emphasized that it is important to identify the risks of deep vein thrombosis and pulmonary embolism (DVT/PE) and to establish that patients can benefit from prophylactic anticoagulation. Patients with hypertension should also be identified because of the implications not only in the cardiovascular and CNS systems but also in the perioperative bleeding. Another important factor is to understand the importance of reducing and treating hypothermia [25].

2.5. Surgery time

The time a patient remains anesthetized is directly related to the frequency of complications; hypothermia, deep venous thrombosis, pulmonary thromboembolism, changes in coagulation, bleeding, alterations in the immune system, and neurovascular compressions are some of the usual drawbacks in prolonged surgery-anesthesia [26]. In plastic surgery, there are procedures that require prolonged times such as patients with combined surgeries and post-bariatric cases with large weight loss. Unfortunately, there is not enough information on these possible complications. Phillips et al. [27] retrospectively studied the relationship between the anesthetic time and the incidence of deleterious effects in 2595 plastic surgery procedures performed under general anesthesia and found that the majority were women with a mean age of 41 years. These authors divided their patients into two groups (less than 4 or more than 4 hours of anesthetic time): nausea and vomiting (2.8 vs. 5.7%, $p = 0.0175$) and urinary retention (0.7 vs. 7.6%, $p < 0.0001$), and 2.5% required reoperations due to surgical complications without statistical differences between the two groups. They had one patient with PE and one with DVT in the group of less than 4 hours of anesthesia. Five (0.19%) were admitted to a hospital for medical or surgical treatment (3 hematomas, 1 PE, and 1 DVT). There were no deaths in this series. Another study of 1200 patients with facial plastic surgery [28] performed under general anesthesia compared the patients with anesthetic time of less than 4 hours (14%) vs. longer anesthesia (86%). There were no catastrophic complications, and the morbidity in 100% of the patients was minimal: one respiratory failure, one patient CNS deficit, one drug allergic reaction, and one patient requiring hospital transfer. There were six cases of prolonged anesthetic recovery time. The incidence of morbidity was similar in both groups. These two studies demonstrated that the time of general anesthesia was not a major determinant in the immediate evolution of these patients operated in ambulatory surgery units.

2.6. Surgeon without anesthesiologist

This is a controversial context where plastic surgeons consider themselves qualified to perform some procedures with local anesthesia and superficial sedation without the presence of an anesthesiologist. Examples to these procedures are variable according to the routines and interests of each surgeon, such as, blepharoplasties, small volume liposuction, coronal and facial rhytidectomies, filler injections, and hair implants, to mention a few. The fact is that each surgical procedure should be properly monitored by the anesthesiologist in charge of patient safety (monitored anesthetic care), and let the surgeon concentrates on his procedures without distracting his attention in monitoring the patient, or administer sedative medications, analgesics, or anesthetics with a very narrow therapeutic window. Although complications are rare, there is no way to predict with certainty when a patient will have a sentinel event or a negative incident, for example, drug toxicity, overdose, drug interaction, hypertensive crisis, anxiety, airway obstruction, and broken heart syndrome, just to mention some of the many possibilities. These are complications that few surgeons are qualified to solve and are part of the anesthesiologist's usual practice. In a series of catastrophic events in ASA 1 and 2 patients, we found a case of death during a ritidoplasty performed without the presence of the anesthesiologist [29]. The frequency of these events is not known, and it is advisable to avoid surgical procedures without the presence of an anesthesiologist, which is classified as negligence.

2.7. The tourist patient

People who travel from one country to another to receive medical attention are called tourist-patients, and their characteristics have different aspects that can modify their risks: cultural traditions, language, common diseases in their region of origin, and physiological adjustments from their recent voyage, especially when being by plane longer than 6 hours. Their preanesthetic evaluation is done shortly after they arrive, and there could be special conditions that are not known by the treating doctors. This type of patient has proliferated in plastic surgery. In our practice, we consider them a management challenge, emphasizing an effective communication that facilitates preoperative assessment, professional care, and a safe return to their place of origin [30].

2.8. Anesthesia technique

The choice of anesthesia method is the responsibility of the anesthesiologist, although patients and surgeons must be aware and consent with the anesthetic plan. In general terms, we can use any kind of anesthesia, although the anesthesiologist should be adapted to factors such as diverse as his/her own experience and knowledge, the characteristics of the surgical unit and the surgeon, the type and duration of surgery, and in particular the characteristics of each patient. It is noteworthy to mention that the *best anesthesia is not the one that is best handled by the anesthesiologist, but the anesthesia procedure that engages better to each patient.* In ambulatory patients, general anesthesia has a preponderant role due to its quick recovery [31], although its immediate side effects are more common when compared to regional anesthesia and have been linked to increased frequency of DVT/PE. When general anesthesia is given, protective ventilation should be used (a tidal volume of 6–8 mL/kg of ideal body weight, less than 30 cm H_2O peak pressure, and PEEP 6–8 cm H_2O), which prevents lung damage, specifically in prolonged surgery.

In our ambulatory and short-stay surgical unit, regional procedures are preferred, especially subarachnoid anesthesia with a lumbar approach for surgeries below T6 segment. We also use spinal anesthesia in some patients with combined surgical procedures up to T4. Single injection of spinal anesthetics and adjuvants is safe, rapid, easy to administer, inexpensive, with a certain degree of postoperative analgesia, and fewer immediate and late residual effects than general anesthesia [32, 33]. We do not use subarachnoid anesthesia with a thoracic approach. In breast, nose, and arm surgeries, we prefer general anesthesia. For facial surgery, we use conscious sedation mixed with local anesthesia [34], and we have just adopted Friedberg's recommendation [35] with propofol or ketofol for facial surgery and sometimes as a sedative complement at the end of spinal anesthesia. The characteristics of propofol make it a safe drug when administered by an anesthesiologist and BIS (60–70) monitoring is recommended, although the Ramsey scale (3–4) can also be used [33, 35].

Monitored anesthesia care is a safe technique in ambulatory and short-stay units. It must be done by an anesthesiologist and goes from simple monitoring of the patient to the use of intravenous drugs and local anesthetics for longer procedures as rejuvenation facial surgery. The most used drugs are propofol, ketamine, midazolam, fentanyl, sufentanil, remifentanil, and dexmedetomidine always supplemented with nasal oxygen [34–39].

Figure 1 shows a schema where the difference between alertness, conscious sedation, deep sedation, and general anesthesia are shown. The vertical line delimits the most relevant clinical data and the appropriate management [34]. Attachment to this scheme is a simple guide to avoid anesthesia complications, especially the airway and cardiovascular and central nervous systems.

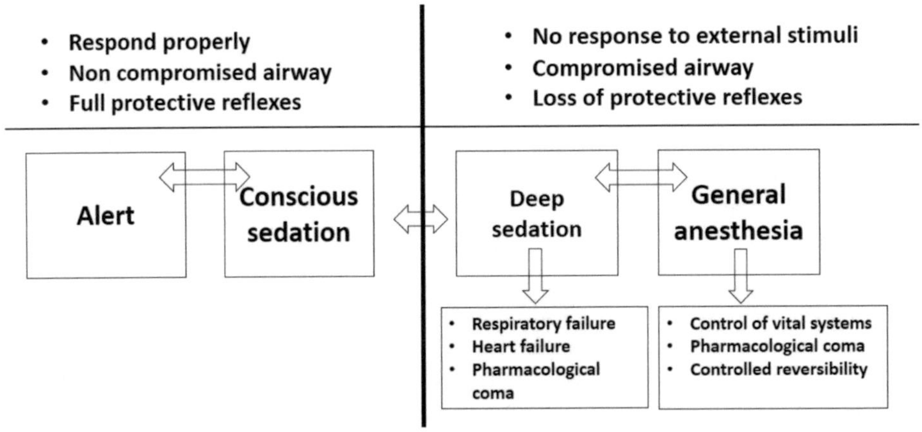

Figure 1. Scheme showing the differences and limits of alertness, conscious sedation, deep sedation, and general anesthesia.

3. Complications

A patient may be complicated by anesthesia, surgery, or a combination of both, for example, infections, venous thrombosis, thromboembolism, bleeding (anemia or hematomas), inadequate scarring, neural damage, overhydration, postoperative emesis, or burns, just to name a few. It is usually impossible to attribute these complications to one single member of the team; therefore, all professionals should function as a teamwork and must share responsibilities as in those patients complicated with DVT/PE. In this chapter, we review the expected complications in anesthesia-plastic surgery and a group of rare incidents that could occur in this clinical setting of which we have observed some.

3.1. Anesthesia complications

Complications of anesthesia can be classified into four different etiological categories: (1) health personnel errors; (2) adverse events to the anesthesia technique; (3) the physical condition of the patients; and (4) sentinel incidents or events. Anesthesia morbidity and mortality rates are approximately the same in countries with a similar life expectancy. The anesthesiologic community of a given country reduces their anesthesia morbidity and mortality data by an acceptable range for their societies using techniques according to their medical culture and historical traditions [40]. Although complications will always exist since erring is human [41], preventive measures are obligatory to reduce complications of anesthesia and to regulate our professional activity to reduce morbidity and mortality statistics [6]. Complications related to anesthesia are rare in plastic surgery, ranging from simple events to catastrophic outcomes, including death.

3.1.1. Unplanned hypothermia

It is the most frequent complication in plastic surgery. Under normal conditions, human thermoregulation mechanisms maintain body temperature from 36.5 to 37.5°C. This homeostasis is achieved by thermoregulatory defense mechanisms such as vasoconstriction, vasodilation, sweating, or chills. Hypothermia is considered when body temperature drops below 36°C. It can occur in the perioperative period; preoperative phase is defined as 1 hour before induction (when patients are prepared for surgery), during the intraoperative phase (total anesthetic time) and postoperative phase (24 postoperative hours) [42, 43]. Unintentional intraoperative decrease in body temperature occurs in a large percentage of surgeries and is secondary to multiple factors. In anesthetized patients, body temperature usually drops 2°C but can drop up to 6°C due to changes done by general anesthesia at the center of thermoregulation, a thermal decrease depending on the dose of the anesthetic. Other important factors of hypothermia are the exposure of the patient to the cold environment of the operating rooms and the failure to actively warm patients. Hypothermia has negative effects such as increased infections, delayed healing, increased intra and postoperative bleeding, increased blood transfusion requirements, increased cardiac morbidity, prolonged duration of anesthetics, and coagulopathies [44, 45]. Therefore, it is necessary to use different methods to avoid it, to reduce its intensity, and to manage it with opportunity; mattresses with forced air or water heating, electrical devices, heating of the intravenous or irrigation solutions, room temperature, and thermal blankets, among others, have shown different degrees of efficacy [46–49].

Some body contouring procedures such as liposuction of various regions, extended or circular abdominoplasty, and multiple surgeries expose body surface in a way that facilitate heat loss. If this is added to the fact that some surgeons are accustomed to utilizing antiseptic solutions in the skin area that will be operated minutes before positioning the patients in the operating table, it accelerates and increases the hypothermia and can be an incident that affects the patient outcome.

Perioperative hypothermia is a complication that must be anticipated, detected early, and treated in a timely manner.

3.1.2. *Toxicity and side effects to drugs*

Side effects to drugs used during anesthesia are sporadic. A background of allergies or hypersensitivity should be investigated at the time of the anesthetic evaluation and avoid its use. Among other drugs, there have been reports of allergies to local anesthetics, muscle relaxants, sugammadex, and propofol, with the most severe reactions to latex. Opioids, especially remifentanil, may induce hyperalgesia. There are undesirable reactions like malignant hyperthermia secondary to halogenated and succinylcholine. These patients must be managed with total intravenous anesthesia or regional anesthesia because local anesthetics are safer and have rarely been associated with this entity [50].

For a couple of decades, local anesthetic toxicity has been the subject of multiple publications. In plastic surgery, there is a controversy over the total doses accepted as safe. Since the original description by Klein [51, 52], various data on safe doses of lidocaine 0.1–0.05% plus epinephrine 1:1,000,000 in tumescent liposuction have been published. Segmental infiltration of reduced lidocaine concentration 0.02% has been used in broader liposuctions [53]. The latest research done in 14 human volunteers has shown that 28 mg/kg without liposuction and 45 mg/kg (dose range 9.2–52 mg/kg.) after liposuction are safe dosages. The authors reported serum lidocaine concentration below levels associated with mild lidocaine systemic toxicity. The probable risk of lidocaine toxicity without liposuction at a dose of 28 mg/kg and with liposuction at a dose of 45 mg/kg was ≤1 per 2000 [54]. Timely diagnosis and management of local anesthetic toxicity with intravenous lipids in severe cases are essential. Lipids in initial dose of 1.5 mL/kg, followed by infusion of 0.25–0.50 mL/kg for 30–60 min. This infusion can be increased if hypotension or asystole persists [55]. After the infusion of iv lipids is stopped, a recurrence of local anesthetics toxicity can happen, so these patients need to be observed for at least 24 hours more.

3.1.3. *Trigeminal cardiac reflex*

Rhinoplasty is a frequent, relatively simple outpatient procedure that can be catastrophically complicated. The trigeminal cardiac reflex is defined as sudden onset of parasympathetic dysrhythmia, bradycardia that can progress to sudden asystole in addition to hypotension, apnea, and gastric hypermotility. This reflex can be initiated with stimulation of the trigeminal nerve during infiltration of the local anesthetic in the nasal columella or during osteotomy [56–59].

3.1.4. Nausea and vomiting

Postoperative emesis is a serious complication in plastic surgery as it may interfere with the results. It occurs after general or neuraxial anesthesia and has been associated with the use of opioids, being more frequent in young women, nonsmokers, and patients with a history of postanesthetic emesis. Prevention is necessary using preoperative medication such as dexamethasone and/or serotonergic antagonists. Metoclopramide has fallen into disuse because of its side effects.

3.1.5. Overhydration

It is associated in tumescent liposuction with large volumes and generous intravenous administration of hydro saline solutions that can induce arterial hypertension, pulmonary edema, and even death.

3.1.6. Deep venous thrombosis and pulmonary thromboembolism

Although these events are not directly attributable to the anesthetic technique, this is one of the factors that may be involved. They are the most feared complications in surgery and are more frequent in liposuction and abdominoplasty [60]. The embolus can be hematic or fatty. The risk factors are young women, contraceptives, air travel of more than 6–8 hours, prolonged surgeries, and thrombophilic pathologies such as factor V Leiden [61, 62]. Preventive measures with elastic stockings and pneumatic compression, early mobilization, antiplatelet agents, heparins, and/or oral anticoagulants are mandatory in high risk patients since this complication is the leading cause of mortality in plastic surgery. In 1,141,418 outpatient surgery procedures, there were 23 fatal events, being the pulmonary embolism the cause in 13 patients. Abdominoplasty was the surgery most commonly associated with death from pulmonary embolism in an office-based surgery facility [63].

3.1.7. Uncommon complications

Most of these types of complications are sentinel incidents that make prevention, diagnosis, and management difficult. The following paragraphs describe some patients seen in our professional practice or referred by colleagues.

3.1.7.1. Postanesthesia-surgery blindness

This entity occurs in ~1:60,000 to 1:125,000 anesthetics procedures and is more frequent in cardiovascular and orthopedic surgery, although there are cases described in plastic surgery [64, 65]. It has been associated with prolonged prone position with the head positioned lower than the thorax, anemia, use of vasoconstrictors, or glycine [66, 67]. Transient or permanent postoperative blindness has also been described following facial injections of fillers as described later.

In our practice, we had a 38-year-old patient who underwent abdominoplasty, liposuction, and fat transfer in her buttocks under spinal-general anesthesia. She developed total blindness manifested in the immediate postanesthetic recovery. MRI showed occipital cortical edema (**Figure 2**), establishing the diagnosis of cortical blindness.

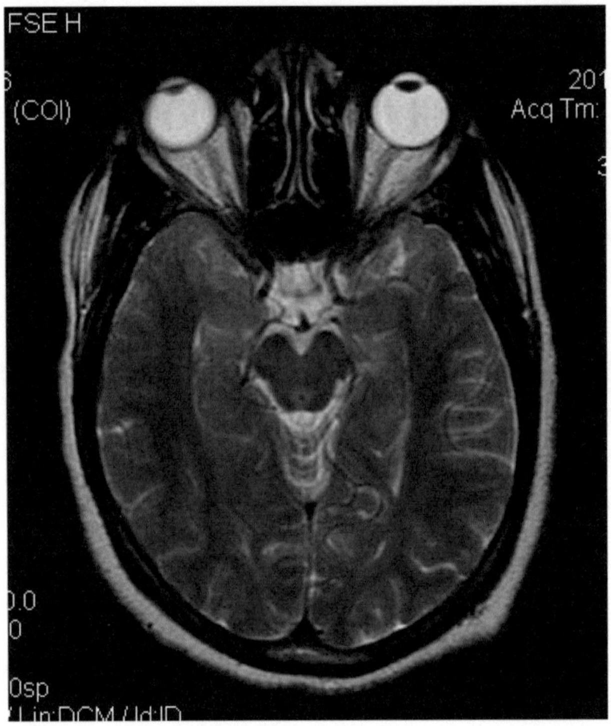

Figure 2. Blindness secondary to cerebral occipital cortical edema.

3.1.7.2. Transient deafness

This rare effect has been reported in subarachnoid anesthesia attributing to sudden changes in endolymph. We had a young patient from Russia who lost her auditory acuity during 5 days after spinal anesthesia for liposuction-gluteal lipoinjection.

3.1.7.3. Broken heart syndrome

Takotsubo's cardiomyopathy or broken heart syndrome is a stress-induced heart disease with sudden left ventricular failure without coronary damage [68]. A young woman developed this syndrome few minutes after nasal infiltration with lidocaine and epinephrine under anesthesia with sevoflurane. The surgery was canceled, and the patient was transferred to a nearby hospital where she was successfully managed.

3.1.7.4. Awakening during general anesthesia

It is a very rare entity with an estimated incidence of 0.1–0.2% but has the potential to cause adverse evolution in the psychological area inducing posttraumatic stress [69]. A 43-year-old patient who underwent transoperative awakening during general anesthesia with enflurane.

3.1.8. *Attempted murder*

Anecdotal situation has been reported on few occasions. We had a case where the spouse tried to assassinate his wife at the end of conscious sedation for rhytidectomy. He injected her with vecuronium, but the timely resuscitation initiated by the recovery area nurse and the clinical suspicion followed to the administration of neostigmine reversed the respiratory failure. The patient was transferred to intensive care unit where the husband made two failed attempts to reinject muscle relaxants.

3.2. Surgical complications

Some surgical complications are listed because of their importance and relation to anesthesia.

3.2.1. *Surgical infections*

Infections are frequent in plastic surgery, from 4% up to 14%, including local infections, blood-borne infections, and distal infections such as pneumonia or infective endocarditis. Breast surgery—implants or reconstructions—body contouring procedures such as liposuction and abdominoplasty, or multiple procedures have been described with more risks of postoperative infections, especially if there are predisposing factors such as diabetes, HIV, cancer, or immunosuppressive treatment. Infections in plastic surgery can be minor due to microbial skin flora to severe cases affected with atypical or multiresistant opportunistic bacteria [70, 71]. The type of infection varies depending on the surgery and the patient. Choice of antibiotics must be meticulous based initially on the clinical suspicion, escalating the antimicrobial when the bacterium is isolated, and its sensitivity is known. The most isolated germs in implant-based reconstruction infections are *Staphylococcus epidermidis, Staphylococcus aureus, Serratia marcescens, Pseudomonas aeruginosa, Enterococcus, Escherichia coli, Enterobacter, Group B streptococcus, Morganella morganii, Propionibacterium,* and *Corynebacterium.* Initial cellulitis can be managed with oral fluoroquinolones. If this treatment fails, intravenous imipenem, gentamicin, and/or vancomycin must be prescribed [72, 73]. Severe infections with methicillin-resistant *Staphylococcus aureus* (MRSA) should be treated aggressively with vancomycin, teicoplanin, or tigecycline, in addition to draining infected sites. Cases with nontuberculous mycobacterial infections are fairly atypical, difficult to diagnose and treat [74–79]. The antimicrobial treatment must be aggressive and prolonged, and when there are implants, these must be removed. **Figure 3** shows a patient infected with *Mycobacterium chelonae* after liposuction.

Necrotizing fasciitis is a rare, potentially fatal, complication in plastic surgery that occurs more in liposuction. It requires extensive, repetitive debridement, and appropriate antimicrobial scheme. The most common germ is *Streptococcus pyogenes* [80].

3.2.2. *Transoperative bleeding and hematoma*

These are uncommon complications, although it does occur in patients undergoing prolonged procedures, especially in the postbariatric ones. A hematoma is present in up to 6% of patients

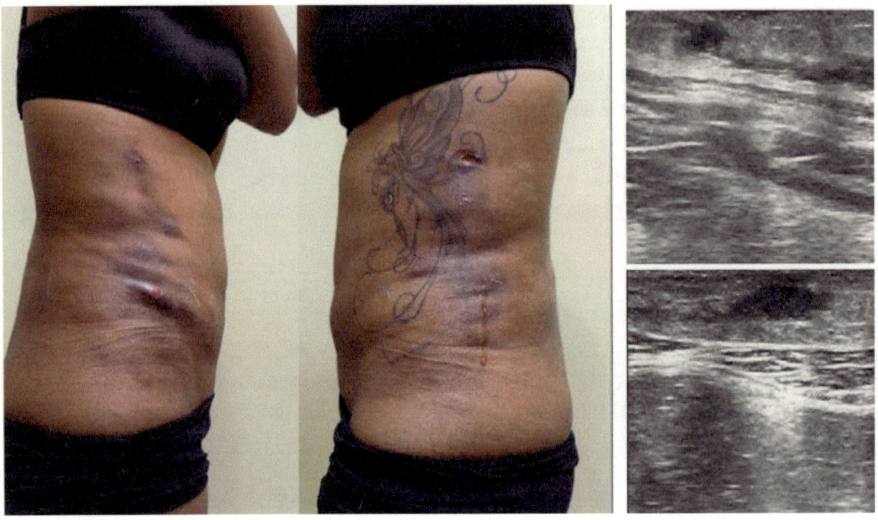

Figure 3. *M. chelonae* after liposuction.

after breast surgery. Facial surgery is rare but compromises long-term results. Most patients are reluctant to hemotransfusion. It is possible to correct moderate anemia without hemodynamic compromise with iron, folic acid, and erythropoietin. **Figure 4** shows typical cases of bleeding that may complicate the definitive outcome of surgery.

3.2.3. Neural damage

Nerve ending injuries are common in liposuction and abdominoplasty and manifest as neuropathic pain. Preventive use of gabapentinoids is useful. Major nerve damage can be seen

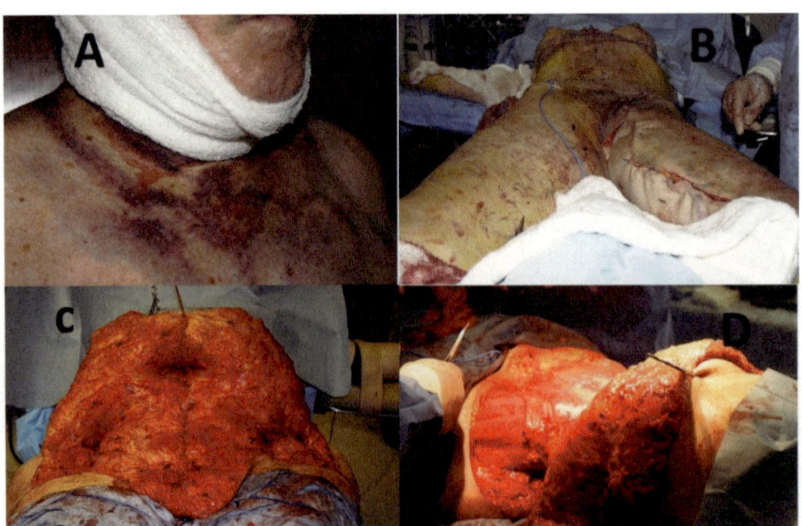

Figure 4. Transoperative active bleeding and residual postsurgical hematomas.

in facial and breast surgery. Inappropriate scarring is an unpredictable risk and sometimes produces neural entrapment with secondary chronic postoperative pain.

3.2.4. Other injuries

Liposuction is one of the procedures that are performed more frequently, and its complications are minimal such as seromas, deformities, and lymphoedema. Serious complications are rare, for example, hematoma (0.15%), pulmonary complications (0.1%), infection (0.1%), and PE (0.06%). When it is combined with other procedures, complication rates are higher. It has also been associated with catastrophic lesions such as pleuropulmonary, abdominal viscera, and vascular damage [81, 82].

3.2.5. Cosmetic filler complications

Soft tissue volumetric augmentation with filler injections is the second most frequent non-surgical procedure performed in plastic surgery, being the face and buttocks the areas more frequently injected. The increased use of a wide range of fillers has shown that they are not harmless, so it is crucial to briefly review possible complications. The transfer of autologous fat in the facial regions is the most used filling substance. There are a great variety of synthetic fillers that can be atoxic and nonimmunogenic or act as a foreign body and induce an immune reaction, granulomas, infections, fibrosis, and long-lasting or permanent body deformities [83–85]. Although very rare, transient or permanent blindness and cerebrovascular emboli are the most devastating complication of forehead and facial injection of synthetic fillers or autologous fat. It is believed that the injected filling can act as a retrograde embolus upon entering the ophthalmic artery or through the normal anastomosis between frontal branch of superficial temporal artery from external carotid artery and supraorbital artery from ophthalmic artery [86]. Cannata et al. [87] described a patient who was injected with polymethylmethacrylate microspheres in the legs, soon after developed infection at the site of injection, followed by postinfectious glomerulonephritis. Kidney biopsy revealed translucent, nonbirefringent microspherical bodies compatible with the injected filler. **Figure 5** shows facial deformations

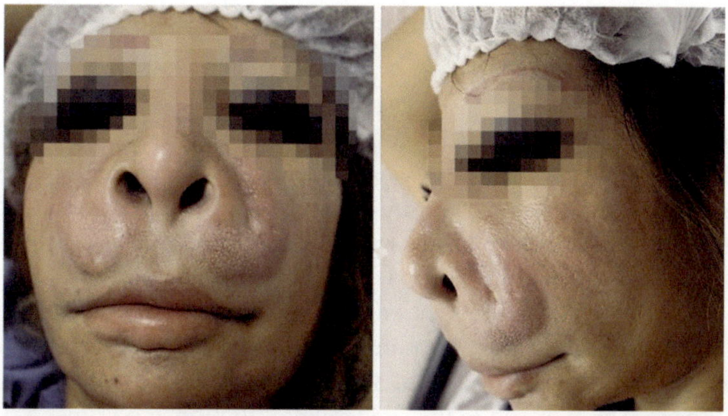

Figure 5. Severe facial deformities secondary to an unknown illegal filler.

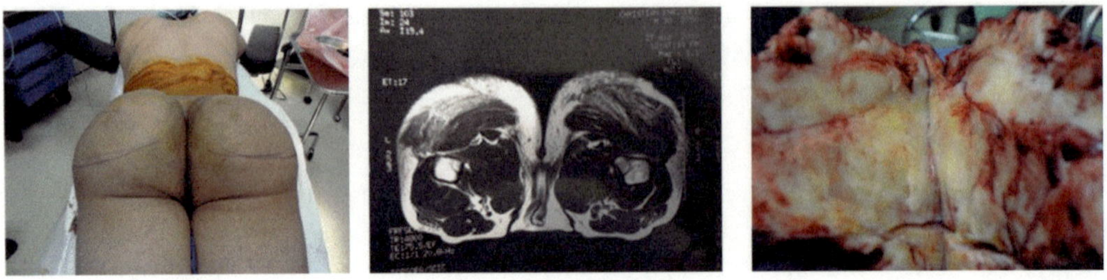

Figure 6. Deformities in the buttocks secondary to unknown substances. Observe extreme fibrosis.

secondary to injection of unknown filler, and **Figure 6** is an MRI that shows fillers injected in the buttocks, which produce fibrosis and deformations of the region by erratic migration, which are very difficult or impossible to correct.

4. Recommendations to reduce complications

Undoubtedly, the meticulous selection of each patient is the key to success in plastic surgery. When a patient does not have a physical and mental state required to undergo plastic surgery, the procedure should be deferred or canceled regardless of the interests of the patient and/or the medical group. When the complexity and risk of the procedure exceed the capacity of the surgical unit and/or the medical group, it is appropriate to refer the patient to a surgical unit or hospital with adequate resources [9, 86–89]. No anesthesia procedure should be considered as a minor method, and it is always necessary to work in a safe and effective surgical facility, following established guidelines, and in permanent communication with surgeons and nurses.

A study conducted in Havana Cuba [90] with 26 patients from that country found that personality traits can determine poor choice of people who apply for cosmetic surgery, some with psychosis and dysmorphophobia that induce expectations higher than the real ones.

5. Legal aspects

We live in a society of litigation where the doctors are easy prey to the ambition of the lawyers and some patients, a society where the governments create groups that exaggerate the rights of the patients making them believe that the improper results of the medical procedures are by negligence. There is a social environment—especially in government hospitals—where physicians are forced to work with multiple deficiencies as a routine practice, where health workers do not have adequate equipment and supplies, with long hours of work and few or no rights at all. There are few and inadequate preventive or curative programs [91]. The syndrome of professional exhaustion (burnout syndrome) has not been considered as a professional disease. To err is human and in this inadequate situation, it becomes a potential threat.

Anesthesiology is a science, with a high risk of undesirable events secondary to the use of drugs and techniques with narrow safety margins that facilitate unexpected complications. On the other hand, plastic surgery is a specialty where the unrealistic high expectations of many patients mean that despite adequate results—surgeons and anesthesiologists can trigger demands—when these results are not what the patient expects, and even when there are no complications. A growing number of patients establish negligence or malpractice claims—justified or not—and our practice tends toward an environment with a high incidence of litigation that sometimes forces specialists to search for geographic areas with a lower incidence of lawsuits [92]. Frequently, decisions of the legal system do not depend on the opinions of medical experts, or medical experts are not properly trained to review the events of a lawsuit in all specialties of medicine and surgery. Patients, their families, and lawyers usually make demands that do not progress due to lack of elements that support malpractice. An attorney should not file a lawsuit without the opinion of a physician skilled in the subject [93].

Park et al.'s [94] study of negligence claims in plastic surgery found responsibility between 30 and 100% of the cases, although the courts recognized that the economic compensation should be adjusted according to the victim, especially when there are associated pathologies which limit and make fairer compensation. Paik et al. [5] reviewed 292 cases of verdicts and liquidation reports in cosmetic breast surgery; the most common lesion was breast disfigurement in 53.1%, and negligent misrepresentation was 98% more likely to be resolved in favor of the complainant, while fraud was 92% more amenable to the complainant. The most common causes of citation were negligence in 88.7% and lack of informed consent in 43.8%. About 58.3% of the cases were in favor of the defendant and 41.7% in favor of the plaintiff. The compensation percentage agreed was 33.4 and 8.3% settlement. Payments ranged from $ 245,000 to $ 300,000 USD. A study with 88 cases of demand found in the west legal database [95] examined facial surgery procedures and found that 62.5% were decided in favor of the surgeon, 9.1% made agreements out of court, and 28.4% went to court for damages due to medical malpractice. The average payment was $ 577,437 USD, and the jury average was $ 352,341 USD, with blepharoplasty and rhytidectomy being the most litigated. In 38.6% of these cases, there were faults in the informed consent. There were also quarrels and disfigurements, functional considerations, and postoperative pain. The authors emphasize the importance of communication between patients and physicians regarding expectations as well as document benefits, alternatives, and specific risks. These studies show that negligence favors the demands in this clinical environment and emphasize that adequate transparency and communication are the key in the doctor-patient relationship, as mentioned in a previous publication [6].

Lawyers have promoted the lawsuit as a part of their modus vivendi. "Have you suffered as a result of a cosmetic procedure that you believe is due to the negligence of the surgeon? If you believe that your surgeon acted negligently and outside of his/her duty to care for you as a patient, we can help you." This type of information is found on the Internet, and it is associated to websites that guide patients on how to formulate their demands. In Colombia, doctors have expressed their concerns about the rigidity of their penal system [96], which temporarily suspended a plastic surgeon, in addition to imposing a prison for less than a year and compensation to the patient for 150,000,000 Colombian pesos (approximately 52,290 USD) in a complicated liposuction with necrotizing fasciitis. The authors discuss different legal, ethical, and surgical, among other topics, and at the end, they argue the possibility to stop practicing surgery due to legal imputations every time a complication occurs. Although this would be an extreme measure, there are many colleagues who have retired after an incident. Well-qualified and experienced anesthesiologists and surgeons are not exempt from perioperative complications.

6. Conclusions

Perioperative complications of patients undergoing plastic surgery are infrequent when the medical group adheres to established guidelines and recommendations. Although these complications cannot be avoided at 100%, it is mandatory to establish preventive programs, and when these events happen, the diagnosis and timely management are imperative. Preanesthetic assessment is mandatory including meticulous search for risk factors; less than 10% of physicians working in the surgical room have disruptive behavior, and up to 98% of clinicians have observing troublesome conduct. It has been mentioned that this inappropriate behavior can facilitate complications. As in hospitals, ambulatory surgery units and all personnel must be properly certified and maintained on a permanent basis [97, 98].

Acknowledgements

We would like to thank the images of www.anestesia-dolor.org for allowing us to publish it.

Conflict of interests

None.

Author details

Víctor M. Whizar-Lugo[1*], Jaime Campos-León[2] and Alejandro Moreno-Guillen[1]

*Address all correspondence to: vwhizar@anestesia-dolor.org

1 Intensive Care Unit, Hospital General de Tijuana, ISESALUD, Tijuana, BC, Mexico

2 Lotus MedGroup, Tijuana, BC, Mexico

References

[1] Domanski MC, Cavale N. Self-reported "worth it" rating of aesthetic surgery in social media. Aesthetic Plastic Surgery. 2012;**36**(6):1292-1295. DOI: 10.1007/s00266-012-9977-z

[2] Mavroforou A, Giannoukas A, Michalodimitrakis E. Medical litigation in cosmetic plastic surgery. Medicine and Law. 2004;**23**(3):479-488

[3] Whizar-Lugo V. Excelencia en anestesia. Rev Cubana de Anestesiología y Reanimación. 2011;**10**(3):176-185

[4] Cima RR, Deschamps C. Role of the surgeon in quality and safety in the operating room environment. General Thoracic and Cardiovascular Surgery. 2013;**61**(1):1-8. DOI: 10.1007/s11748-012-0111-6

[5] Paik AM, Mady LJ, Sood A, Eloy JA, Lee ES. A look inside the courtroom: An analysis of 292 cosmetic breast surgery medical malpractice cases. Aesthetic Surgery Journal. 2014;**34**(1):79-86. DOI: 10.1177/1090820X13515702

[6] Whizar-Lugo V. Prevención en anestesiología. Anest Mex. 2009;**21**(2):118-138

[7] Ersek RA. Office-based plastic surgery. Seminars in Plastic Surgery. 2007;**21**(2):115-122. DOI: 10.1055/s-2007-979212

[8] Hunstad JP, Walk PH. Office-based anesthesia. Seminars in Plastic Surgery. 2007;**21**(2): 103-107. DOI: 10.1055/s-2007-979210

[9] Van De Velde M, Kuypers M, Teunkens A, Devroe S. Risk and safety of anesthesia outside the operating room. Minerva Anestesiologica. 2009;**75**(5):345-348

[10] Deckert D, Zecha-Stallinger A, Haas T, von Goedecke A, Lederer W, Wenzel V. Anesthesia outside the core operating area. Der Anaesthesist. 2007;**56**(10):1028-1037

[11] Missant C, Van de Velde M. Morbidity and mortality related to anaesthesia outside the operating room. Current Opinion in Anaesthesiology. 2004;**17**(4):323-327. DOI: 10.1097/01.aco.0000137091.75602.34

[12] Rosenberg NM, Urman RD, Gallagher S, Stenglein J, Liu X, Shapiro FE. Effect of an office-based surgical safety system on patient outcomes. Eplasty. 2012;**12**:e59

[13] Katz JD. Control of the environment in the operating room. Anesthesia and Analgesia. 2017;**125**(4):1214-1218. DOI: 10.1213/ANE.0000000000001626

[14] Shapiro FE, Pawlowski JB, Rosenberg NM, Liu X, Feinstein DM, Urman RD. The use of in-situ simulation to improve safety in the plastic surgery office: A feasibility study. Eplasty. 2014;**14**:e2

[15] Starling J 3rd, Thosani MK, Coldiron BM. Determining the safety of office-based surgery: What 10 years of Florida data and 6 years of Alabama data reveal. Dermatologic Surgery. 2012;**38**(2):171-177. DOI: 10.1111/j.1524-4725.2011.02206.x

[16] Bruce J, Russell EM, Mollison J, Krukowski ZH. The measurement and monitoring of surgical adverse events. Health Technology Assessment. 2001;**5**(22):1-194

[17] http://www.cofepris.gob.mx/AS/Documents/COMISI%C3%93N%20DE%20OPERACI%C3%93N%20SANITARIA_Documentos%20para%20publicar%20en%20la%20secci%C3%B3n%20de%20MEDICAMENTOS/Alertas/27022015.pdf [Accessed: Jul 20, 2017]

[18] Salisbury M. Certification for office-based plastic surgery. Seminars in Plastic Surgery. 2007;**21**(2):133-134. DOI: 10.1055/s-2007-979215

[19] Ellsworth WA, Basu CB, Iverson RE. Perioperative considerations for patient safety during cosmetic surgery—Preventing complications. The Canadian Journal of Plastic Surgery. 2009;**17**(1):9-16

[20] Poore SO, Sillah NM, Mahajan AY, Gutowski KA. Patient safety in the operating room: I. Preoperative. Plastic and Reconstructive Surgery. 2012;**130**(5):1038-1047. DOI: 10.1097/PRS.0b013e31826945d6

[21] Poore SO, Sillah NM, Mahajan AY, Gutowski KA. Patient safety in the operating room: II. Intraoperative and postoperative. Plastic and Reconstructive Surgery. 2012;**130**(5):1048-1058. DOI: 10.1097/PRS.0b013e318267d531

[22] Collins SJ, Newhouse R, Porter J, Talsma A. Effectiveness of the surgical safety checklist in correcting errors: A literature review applying Reason's Swiss cheese model. AORN Journal. 2014;**100**(1):65-79.e5. DOI: 10.1016/j.aorn.2013.07.024

[23] Pugel AE, Simianu VV, Flum DR, Patchen Dellinger E. Use of the surgical safety checklist to improve communication and reduce complications. Journal of Infection and Public Health. 2015;**8**(3):219-225. DOI: 10.1016/j.jiph.2015.01.001

[24] Walker A, Reshamwalla S, Wilson IH. Surgical safety checklists: Do they improve outcomes? British Journal of Anaesthesia. 2012;**109**(1):47-54. DOI: 10.1093/bja/aes175

[25] Trussler AP, Tabbal GN. Patient safety in plastic surgery. Plastic and Reconstructive Surgery. 2012;**130**(3):470e-478e. DOI: 10.1097/PRS.0b013e31825dc349

[26] Kodra N, Shpata V, Ohri I. Risk factors for postoperative pulmonary complications after abdominal surgery. Open Access Macedonian Journal of Medical Sciences. 2016;**4**(2):259-263. DOI: 10.3889/oamjms.2016.059

[27] Phillips BT, Wang ED, Rodman AJ, Watterson PA, Smith KL, Finical SJ, et al. Anesthesia duration as a marker for surgical complications in office-based plastic surgery. Annals of Plastic Surgery. 2012;**69**(4):408-411. DOI: 10.1097/SAP.0b013e31825f4e5a

[28] Gordon NA, Koch ME. Duration of anesthesia as an indicator of morbidity and mortality in office-based facial plastic surgery: A review of 1200 consecutive cases. Archives of Facial Plastic Surgery. 2006;**8**(1):47-53. DOI: 10.1001/archfaci.8.1.47

[29] Whizar-Lugo VM, Cisneros-Corral R, Maldonado Romero JA. Muerte o daño neural por anestesia en pacientes de bajo riesgo. Análisis de 25 casos y del impacto a largo plazo en los anestesiólogos. Anest Mex. 2007;**19**(1):88-98

[30] Whizar-Lugo V, Flores-Carrillo JC, Campos-León J, Parra-Beltrán P, Azamar-Llamas D. Perioperative care of tourist-patients. Journal of Anesthesia and Critical Care: Open Access. 2015;**3**(4):00119. DOI: 10.15406/jaccoa.2015.03.00119

[31] Spring MA, Stoker DA, Holloway J, Weintraub M, Stevens WG. Office-based plastic surgery with general anesthesia: Efficiency of cost and time. Seminars in Plastic Surgery. 2007;**21**(2):99-101. DOI: 10.1055/s-2007-979209

[32] Whizar LV, Flores CJC, Campos LJ, Silva V. Spinal anaesthesia for ambulatory and short-stay plastic surgery procedures. In: Whizar LV, editor. Topics in Spinal Anaesthesia. Croatia: InTech; 2014. pp. 39-66. DOI: 10.5772/58407

[33] Whizar-Lugo VM, Cisneros-Corral R, Reyes-Aveleyra MA, Campos-León J, Shakhov A. Anestesia subaracnoidea en cirugía plástica ambulatoria. Anest Mex. 2008;**20**(1):23-33

[34] Whizar LV, Cisneros CR, Reyes AMA, Campos LJ. Anestesia para cirugía facial cosmética. Anest Mex. 2005;**17**(3):117-131

[35] Friedberg BL. Propofol in office-based plastic surgery. Seminars in Plastic Surgery. 2007; **21**(2):129-132. DOI: 10.1055/s-2007-979214

[36] Girling VRG, Salisbury M. Sedation monitor for the office-based plastic surgery setting. Seminars in Plastic Surgery. 2007;**21**(2):123-128. DOI: 10.1055/s-2007-979213

[37] Bitar G, Mullis W, Jacobs W, Matthews D, Beasley M, Smith K, et al. Safety and efficacy of office-based surgery with monitored anesthesia care/sedation in 4778 consecutive plastic surgery procedures. Plastic and Reconstructive Surgery. 2003;**111**(1):150-156. DOI: 10.1097/01.PRS.0000037756.88297.BC

[38] Failey C, Aburto J, de la Portilla HG, Romero JF, Lapuerta L, Barrera A. Office-based outpatient plastic surgery utilizing total intravenous anesthesia. Aesthetic Surgery Journal. 2013;**33**(2):270-274. DOI: 10.1177/1090820X12472694

[39] Hasen KV, Samartzis D, Casas LA, Mustoe TA. An outcome study comparing intravenous sedation with midazolam/fentanyl (conscious sedation) versus propofol infusion (deep sedation) for aesthetic surgery. Plastic and Reconstructive Surgery. 2003;**112**(6):1683-1689

[40] Cooper JB, Davies JM, Desmonts JM, Lun JL, Crul JF, Pierce EC, et al. Conference report. 1986 Meeting of international committee for prevention of anesthesia mortality and morbidity. Canadian Journal of Anaesthesia. 1988;**35**(3):287-293

[41] Detmer DE. Erring is human: Will we cross the quality chasm? Quall. 2001;**10**(2):68-69

[42] Sessler DI. Temperature monitoring and perioperative thermoregulation. Anesthesiology. 2008;**109**(2):318-338. DOI: 10.1097/ALN.0b013e31817f6d76

[43] Evans GR, Scholz T, Brandt K. Outpatient surgery. Plastic and Reconstructive Surgery. 2015;**136**(1):89e-95e. DOI: 10.1097/PRS.0000000000001335

[44] Lenhardt R. The effect of anesthesia on body temperature control. Frontiers in Bioscience (Scholar Edition). 2010;**2**:1145-1154

[45] Horosz B, Malec-Milewska M. Inadvertent intraoperative hypothermia. Anaesthesiology Intensive Therapy. 2013;**45**(1):38-43. DOI: 10.5603/AIT.2013.0009

[46] Madrid E, Urrútia G, Roqué i Figuls M, Pardo-Hernandez H, Campos JM, Paniagua P, et al. Active body surface warming systems for preventing complications caused by inadvertent perioperative hypothermia in adults. Cochrane Database of Systematic Reviews. 2016;**4**:CD009016. DOI: 10.1002/14651858.CD009016.pub2

[47] John M, Ford J, Harper M. Peri-operative warming devices: Performance and clinical application. Anaesthesia. 2014;**69**(6):623-638. DOI: 10.1111/anae.12626

[48] Horosz B, Malec-Milewska M. Methods to prevent intraoperative hypothermia. Anaesthesiology Intensive Therapy. 2014;**46**(2):96-100. DOI: 10.5603/AIT.2014.0019

[49] Bindu B, Bindra A, Rath G. Temperature management under general anesthesia: Compulsion or option. Journal of Anaesthesiology Clinical Pharmacology. 2017;**33**(3):306-316. DOI: 10.4103/joacp.JOACP_334_16

[50] Whizar-Lugo VM, Cisneros-Corral R, Campos-León J, Carrillo-Flores JC. Spinal ropivacaine is safe in malignant hyperthermia. A case report. Anest Mex. 2004;**16**(4):227-230

[51] Klein JA. Anesthesia for liposuction in dermatologic surgery. The Journal of Dermatologic Surgery and Oncology. 1988;**14**(10):1124-1132

[52] Klein JA. Tumescent technique for regional anesthesia permits lidocaine doses of 35 mg/kg for liposuction. The Journal of Dermatologic Surgery and Oncology. 1990;**16**(3):248-263

[53] Wang G, Cao WG, Li SL, Liu LN, Jiang ZH. Safe extensive tumescent liposuction with segmental infiltration of lower concentration lidocaine under monitored anesthesia care. Annals of Plastic Surgery. 2015;**74**(1):6-11. DOI: 10.1097/SAP.0b013e3182933de7

[54] Klein JA, Jeske DR. Estimated maximal safe dosages of tumescent lidocaine. Anesthesia and Analgesia. 2016;**122**(5):1350-1359. DOI: 10.1213/ANE.0000000000001119

[55] Whizar-Lugo VM. Tratamiento de la toxicidad por anestésicos locales. Uso de lípidos intravenosos. Anest Mex. 2009;**21**(1):73-76

[56] Meuwly C, Chowdhury T, Sandu N, Reck M, Erne P, Schaller B. Anesthetic influence on occurrence and treatment of the trigemino-cardiac reflex: A systematic literature review. Medicine (Baltimore). 2015;**94**(18):e807. DOI: 10.1097/MD.0000000000000807

[57] Chowdhury T, Mendelowith D, Golanov E, Spiriev T, Arasho B, Sandu N, et al. Trigeminocardiac reflex: The current clinical and physiological knowledge. Journal of Neurosurgical Anesthesiology. 2015;**27**(2):136-147. DOI: 10.1097/ANA.0000000000000065

[58] Özçelik D, Toplu G, Türkseven A, Sezen G, Ankarali H. The importance of the trigeminal cardiac reflex in rhinoplasty surgery. Annals of Plastic Surgery. 2015;**75**(2):213-218. DOI: 10.1097/SAP.0000000000000061

[59] Yorgancilar E, Gun R, Yildirim M, Bakir S, Akkus Z, Topcu I. Determination of trigeminocardiac reflex during rhinoplasty. International Journal of Oral and Maxillofacial Surgery. 2012;**41**(3):389-393. DOI: 10.1016/j.ijom.2011.12.025

[60] Nath SS, Roy D, Ansari F, Pawar ST. Anaesthetic complications in plastic surgery. Indian Journal of Plastic Surgery. 2013;**46**(2):445-452. DOI: 10.4103/0970-0358.118626

[61] Whizar-Lugo VM, Cisneros-Corral R. Factor V Leiden y anestesia. Informe de dos pacientes. Anest Mex. 2008;**20**(2):98-101

[62] Whizar-Lugo VM, Hurtado Muñoz R. Factor V de Leiden y anestesia. Anest Mex. 2008; **20**(3):122-131

[63] Keyes GR, Singer R, Iverson RE, McGuire M, Yates J, Gold A, et al. Mortality in outpatient surgery. Plastic and Reconstructive Surgery. 2008;**122**(1):245-250. DOI: 10.1097/PRS.0b013e31817747fd

[64] Moura FC, Cunha LP, Monteiro ML. Bilateral visual loss after liposuction: Case report and review of the literature. Clinics (São Paulo, Brazil). 2006;**61**(5):489-491. DOI: org/10.1590/S1807-59322006000500018

[65] Foroozan R, Varon J. Bilateral anterior ischemic optic neuropathy after liposuction. Journal of Neuro-Ophthalmology. 2004;**24**(3):211-213

[66] Roth S, Thisted RA, Erickson JP, Black S, Schreider BD. Eye injuries after non-ocular surgery: A study of 60,965 anaesthetics from 1988 to 1992. Anesthesiology. 1996;**85**:1020-1027

[67] Warner ME, Warner MA, Garrity JA. The frequency of perioperative vision loss. Anesthesia and Analgesia. 2001;**93**:1417-1421

[68] Rodrigues LB, Batista A, Monteiro F, Duarte JS. ST-segment elevation during general anesthesia for non-cardiac surgery: A case of takotsubo. Brazilian Journal of Anesthesiology. 2015;**65**(5):403-406. DOI: 10.1016/j.bjane.2014.11.005

[69] Laukkala T, Ranta S, Wennervirta J, Henriksson M, Suominen K, Hynynen M. Long-term psychosocial outcomes after intraoperative awareness with recall. Anesthesia and Analgesia. 2014;**119**(1):86-92. DOI: 10.1213/ANE.0000000000000257

[70] Long C, Sue GR, Chattopadhyay A, Huis In't Veld E, Lee GK. Critical evaluation of risk factors of infection following 2-stage implant-based breast reconstruction. Plastic and Reconstructive Surgery-Global Open 2017;**5**(7):e1386. DOI: 10.1097/GOX.0000000000001386

[71] Wong SS, Wong SC, Yuen KY. Infections associated with body modification. Journal of the Formosan Medical Association. 2012;**111**(12):667-681. DOI: 10.1016/j.jfma.2012.10.016

[72] Cohen JB, Carroll C, Tenenbaum MM, Myckatyn TM. Breast implant-associated infections: The role of the National Surgical Quality Improvement Program and the local microbiome. Plastic and Reconstructive Surgery. 2015;**136**(5):921-929. DOI: 10.1097/PRS.0000000000001682

[73] Weichman KE, Levine SM, Wilson SC, Choi M, Karp NS. Antibiotic selection for the treatment of infectious complications of implant-based breast reconstruction. Annals of Plastic Surgery. 2013;**71**(2):140-143. DOI: 10.1097/SAP.0b013e3182590924

[74] Brown-Elliott BA, Philley JV. Rapidly growing mycobacteria. Microbiology Spectrum. 2017;**5**(1):5-6. DOI: 10.1128/microbiolspec.TNMI7-0027-2016

[75] Nagao M, Sonobe M, Bando T, Saito T, Shirano M, Matsushima A, et al. Surgical site infection due to *Mycobacterium peregrinum*: A case report and literature review. International Journal of Infectious Diseases. 2009;**13**(2):209-211. DOI: 10.1016/j.ijid.2008.06.018

[76] Vinh DC, Rendina A, Turner R, Embil JM. Breast implant infection with *Mycobacterium fortuitum* group: Report of case and review. The Journal of Infection. 2006;**52**(3):e63-e67. DOI: 10.1016/j.jinf.2005.07.004

[77] Rivera-Olivero IA, Guevara A, Escalona A, Oliver M, Pérez-Alfonzo R, Piquero J, et al. Soft-tissue infections due to non-tuberculous mycobacteria following mesotherapy. What is the price of beauty. Enfermedades Infecciosas y Microbiología Clínica. 2006; **24**(5):302-306

[78] Lizaso D, García M, Aguirre A, Esposto A. Infección protésica mamaria por *Mycobacterium fortuitum* en una paciente con lupus eritematoso sistémico. Revista Chilena de Infectología. 2011;**28**(5):474-478. DOI: /S0716-10182011000600013

[79] Hammond SE, Al-Bayati A, Joumblat N, Salgado CJ. *Mycobacterium chelonae* infection of the buttocks secondary to lipofilling: A case report and review of the literature. Aesthetic Plastic Surgery. 2017;**41**(5):1150-1154. DOI: 10.1007/s00266-017-0890-3

[80] Marchesi A, Marcelli S, Parodi PC, Perrotta RE, Riccio M, Vaienti L. Necrotizing fasciitis in aesthetic surgery: A review of the literature. Aesthetic Plastic Surgery. 2017;**41**(2): 352-358. DOI: 10.1007/s00266-016-0754-2

[81] Kaoutzanis C, Gupta V, Winocour J, Layliev J, Ramirez R, Grotting JC, et al. Cosmetic liposuction: Preoperative risk factors, major complication rates, and safety of combined procedures. Aesthetic Surgery Journal. 2017;**37**(6):680-694. DOI: 10.1093/asj/sjw243

[82] You JS, Chung YE, Baek SE, Chung SP, Kim MJ. Imaging findings of liposuction with an emphasis on postsurgical complications. Korean Journal of Radiology. 2015;**16**(6): 1197-1206. DOI: 10.3348/kjr.2015.16.6.1197

[83] Szantyr A, Orski M, Marchewka I, Szuta M, Orska M, Zapała J. Ocular complications following autologous fat injections into facial area: Case report of a recovery from visual loss after ophthalmic artery occlusion and a review of the literature. Aesthetic Plastic Surgery. 2017;**41**(3):580-584. DOI: 10.1007/s00266-017-0805-3

[84] Prado G, Rodríguez-Feliz J. Ocular pain and impending blindness during facial cosmetic injections: Is your office prepared? Aesthetic Plastic Surgery. 2017;**41**(1):199-203. DOI: 10.1007/s00266-016-0728-4

[85] Chou CC, Chen HH, Tsai YY, Li YL, Lin HJ. Choroid vascular occlusion and ischemic optic neuropathy after facial calcium hydroxyapatite injection—A case report. BMC Surgery. 2015;**15**:21. DOI: 10.1186/s12893-015-0007-3

[86] Li X, Du L, Lu JJ. A novel hypothesis of visual loss secondary to cosmetic facial filler injection. Annals of Plastic Surgery. 2015;**75**(3):258-260. DOI: 10.1097/SAP.0000000000000572

[87] Cannata-Ortiz P, Gracia C, Aouad Y, Barat A, Martinez-Gonzalez MA, Rossello G, et al. Small vessel microembolization and acute glomerulonephritis following infection of aesthetic filler implants. Diagnostic Pathology. 2016;**11**:2. DOI: 10.1186/s13000-016-0453-y

[88] Nekhendzy V, Ramaiah VK. Prevention of perioperative and anesthesia-related complications in facial cosmetic surgery. Facial Plastic Surgery Clinics of North America. 2013;**21**(4):559-577. DOI: 10.1016/j.fsc.2013.07.011

[89] Robbertze R, Posner KL, Domino KB. Closed claims review of anesthesia for procedures outside the operating room. Current Opinion in Anaesthesiology. 2006;**19**(4):436-442. DOI: 10.1097/01.aco.0000236146.46346.fe

[90] Abreu de la Torre C, Francis TO, Alessandrini GR, Macías BR, Leal E. Perfil de personalidad en pacientes que solicitan cirugía estética. Cirugía Plástica. 2000;**10**(3):97-101

[91] Gupta N, Garg R. Professional burnout in anaesthesia and critical care—How to decrease it. Journal of Anesthesia and Critical Care: Open Access. 2015;**2**(3):00056. DOI: 10.15406/jaccoa.2015.02.00056

[92] Kaplan JL, Hammert WC, Zin JE. Lawsuits against plastic surgeons: Does locale affect incidence of claims? The Canadian Journal of Plastic Surgery. 2007;**15**(3):155-157

[93] Horton JB, Reece E, Janis JE, Broughton G 2nd, Hollier L, Thornton JF, et al. Expert witness reform. Plastic and Reconstructive Surgery. 2007;**120**(7):2095-2100. DOI: 10.1097/01.prs.0000296049.42259.39

[94] Park BY, Pak JH, Hong SE, Kang SR. The legal doctrine on 'Limitation of liability' in the precedent analysis on plastic surgery medical malpractice lawsuits. Journal of Korean Medical Science. 2015;**30**(12):1718-1722. DOI: 10.3346/jkms.2015.30.12.1718

[95] Svider PF, Keeley BR, Zumba O, Mauro AC, Setzen M, Eloy JA. From the operating room to the courtroom: A comprehensive characterization of litigation related to facial plastic surgery procedures. The Laryngoscope. 2013;**123**(8):1849-1853. DOI: 10.1002/lary.23905

[96] Guzmán F, Arias CA, Moreno SE. El ejercicio de la cirugía se encuentra en peligro, a propósito de la sentencia N° 33.920 de la Honorable Corte Suprema de Justicia sobre la condena a cirujano plástico de Cali. Revista Colombiana de Cirugía. 2012;**27**:99-113

[97] Villafranca A, Hamlin C, Enns S, Jacobsohn E. Disruptive behaviour in the perioperative setting: A contemporary review. Canadian Journal of Anaesthesia. 2017;**64**(2):128-140. DOI: 10.1007/s12630-016-0784-x

[98] Melloni C. Anesthesia and sedation outside the operating room: How to prevent risk and maintain good quality. Current Opinion in Anaesthesiology. 2007;**20**(6):513-519. DOI: 10.1097/ACO.0b013e3282f06ba6